Pr
Essential Strategies fc

Tami Anastasia comes to the rescue of stressed out and burned out caregivers. *Essential Strategies for the Dementia Caregiver* encourages caregivers to feel their feelings, find workarounds through trial and error, and discover both the joy and sorrow in the caregiving journey.

— **Denise Rousset, Publisher, Sentinel Newspapers**

Tami Anastasia's PACE framework - permission, acknowledgment, compassion, empowerment - gives caregivers permission to be human. Anastasia's own compassion shines through as she delivers advice and action plans designed to ease the caregiver's burden.

— **Maria Nicolacoudis, MA, CEO
Hearts & Minds Activity Center**

At last! *Essential Strategies for the Dementia Caregiver* provides a game plan for each challenging dementia behavior. Anastasia's easy-to-follow formula is a gamechanger for dementia caregivers.

— **Joan McCreary, CPO® Owner, JMPO**

Essential Strategies for the Dementia Caregiver is the one book every dementia caregiver needs. Its straightforward approach provides practical solutions to common challenges, while also addressing the nuances of family dynamics, loss, and love.

— **Dedra Jize, OT, CSA Geriatric Care Manager**

Essential Strategies for the Dementia Caregiver is proof that Tami Anastasia is willing to have the hard conversations. Drawing on her decades of experience as a dementia counselor and consultant, Anastasia tackles everything from taking away driving privileges to caregiver resentment. This book provides the roadmap every caregiver needs.

— **Vicki Ratner, M.D.**

This is the book every caregiver should have within arm's reach. Anastasia's down-to-earth, practical advice provides the support and strategies dementia caregivers need.

— **Jim McCabe, Ph.D.**

Essential Strategies for the Dementia Caregiver will make dementia caregivers feel heard and understood. Infused with compassion and chock-full of advice, Anastasia's book reassures caregivers that they are not alone, that taking care of themselves is as important as taking care of their loved ones, and that they are appreciated.

— **Paula Marks, Vice President of Care Partnerships**

Essential Strategies for the
Dementia Caregiver

Learning to PACE Yourself

Tami Anastasia, MA

Essential Strategies for the Dementia Caregiver: Learning to PACE Yourself
by Tami Anastasia, MA

Copyright © 2022 Tami Anastasia

All rights reserved. No portion of this book may be reproduced in any form without permission from the publisher, except as permitted by U.S. copyright law. For permissions contact: tami@tamianastasia.com

Cover design and illustrations by Sandy Holtzscher
Page design by Robert Henry, righthandpublishing.com

Published by Tami Anastasia
P.O. Box 320672, Los Gatos, CA 95032
Visit the author's website at tamianastasia.com

ISBN: 979-8-9853153-0-1

Printed in the USA

First Edition

To my Grammy A.
and to all of the caregivers who
have invited me to be a part of their journey

Foreword

The dementia caregiving journey is alternately perplexing, demanding, and rewarding. Without a roadmap, the path is fraught with seemingly insurmountable obstacles — hurtful words, behaviors that don't make sense, and gradually increasing grief. In *Essential Strategies for the Dementia Caregiver: Learning to PACE Yourself,* Tami Anastasia provides both a roadmap and a compass, helping to ensure you'll find a way forward.

That compass would have been helpful for Virginia (Ginny) and me, and might have prevented enormous frustration and heartache. She and I met on a dance floor in 1982, and I fell hard for the vivacious New Yorker of Italian heritage who greeted everyone with a warm, broad smile. Yet after building a life together for over two decades, I could no longer find the woman who captured my heart. She became caustic, accusatory, and impossible to live with — so much so that I rented a storage locker and packed most of my belongings.

Still, I wasn't ready to throw in the towel, and I think we both wanted to make our marriage work. Ginny agreed to marriage counseling, but after about six months, the counselor pulled me aside and said, "Something is going on, but I can't put my finger on it." Though Ginny and I continued seeking help, our relationship remained on the rocks.

The "I can't put my finger on it" feeling is familiar to care partners whose loved ones haven't yet been diagnosed with dementia. My lightbulb moment came after an outing to our favorite Indian restaurant. Ginny became suspicious when I greeted the hostess by name. Insisting that she'd never eaten there, Ginny was convinced I knew the hostess because I'd taken another woman to the restaurant. She was unwavering in her belief even when I showed her the credit card receipts from our previous meals. Although I didn't understand what was happening, I knew that Ginny's response was rooted in something more than marital discord.

Thus began Ginny's medical odyssey. Our doctor weighed in, saying that maybe Ginny was simply getting older and experiencing normal memory loss. But, as the months went by, I recorded many personality changes, along with behavioral and language issues. That was a list the doctor couldn't ignore. A referral to a neurologist led to additional tests but no real answers.

A decade later, I began to think that certain events within a short timespan may have conspired to put Ginny at greater risk for dementia. Her car was T-boned, resulting in a hard knock to the head, plastic surgery to retrieve pieces of glass from her face, and months of healing. That type of head injury likely wasn't her first, as she'd previously been a ski patroller and had donned rollerblades a time or two. On top of that, months later, Ginny underwent hours of anesthesia for back surgery. While she was recovering, we watched in horror as the Twin Towers fell on September 11, knowing that our friend, Muriel, was likely reporting to work there around that time. Her body was never found. I believe that this pile-on of events, and more, may have had a lasting impact on her brain. I'll never know for sure.

I kept pushing for answers. Ultimately, we were referred to a teaching hospital and center of excellence for dementia, where Ginny received their best-guess diagnosis. At the time, there were fewer diagnostic tests available than today. I was unprepared for years of caregiving, yet also felt out of place in various support groups I tried. I was frustrated that I couldn't find simple answers to my seemingly simple questions. But I was determined to learn, and that gave me the understanding and resources to make the best life possible for us both. I was surprised to learn along the way that dementia isn't a disease; it's actually a syndrome caused by one or more diseases, disorders, or conditions.

In the last year of Ginny's life, I decided to retire early to spend more time at her side and establish the Dementia Society of America®. Our primary goal is to educate the public about this widespread syndrome and to support the individuals living with dementia and the families, friends, and professionals who care for them. In addition, we provide non-medical grants for music, art, movement, and tactile stimulation programs, as well as recognition for outstanding innovation, research, and care.

Our mission aligns with the book you're holding. Because Tami takes a holistic view of dementia, you'll undoubtedly find your spot on the roadmap she provides. Tami works with care partners daily to provide plans and tools to tackle today's challenges while planning for the future. In *Essential Strategies for the Dementia Caregiver*, she utilizes her PACE framework to share with readers the strategies she uses with her counseling clients and support group attendees. You may see yourself within the vignettes of fictional families, find yourself turning to a worksheet to record your observations, or quickly flipping to the 4 D's of Dementia Care when your loved one is shadowing or argumentative. Wherever you are on your caregiving journey, you will discover knowledge and comfort within these pages.

Kevin Jameson
Founder, President, CEO, and Volunteer
Dementia Society of America

Kevin Jameson is the founder of the Dementia Society of America, a nationwide, volunteer-driven nonprofit organization dedicated to increasing dementia awareness and serving all those affected.

Table of Contents

PREFACE 1

INTRODUCTION 3

PART I. DEMENTIA BASICS 6

    Defining Dementia 6

    The Brain and Dementia 10

    How Dementia Affects Your Loved One 12

    Stages of Dementia 16

    What Your Loved One Needs from You 18

    Action Plan: Knowledge is Power 22

PART II. SURVIVING THE CAREGIVER JOURNEY: PACE YOURSELF 23

    PACE: P = Permission for Trial and Error 25

        Developing Patience 27

        Providing Structure 32

        Action Plan: Nurturing Your Patience 35

    PACE: A = Acknowledge Their Reality 36

        Understanding Their World 36

        Reliving Past Trauma 41

        Responding to Your Loved One 42

        Empathetic Responses 46

    Distracting with Activities 49

    Action Plan: Response Preparedness 55

PACE: C = Compassionate Care 56

    Having the Conversation About Dementia Care Options 56

    Communicating with Kindness 61

    Having Compassion for Yourself 71

    Feeling Unappreciated and Resentful 77

    Dealing with Loss, Sadness, and Grief 83

    Ambiguous Loss and Anticipatory Grief 88

    The Role of a Support Network 92

    Caregiver Guilt 103

    Compassionate Self-Understanding 109

    PACE Caregiver Principles 113

    Action Plan: Understanding Your Feelings 115

PACE: E = Empower Yourself 117

    Educating Yourself 117

    Dealing with Other Family Members 128

    Establishing an Emergency Plan 140

    Hiring In-Home Care 142

    Placement 154

    Transitioning into a Care Community 162

    Hospice Care 170

    Bereavement 176

    Action Plan: Paving the Way 181

Part III. The 4 D's of Dementia Care 182

- Repetitive Questions 184
- Bathing 190
- Toileting 198
- Incontinence 203
- Apathy 208
- Anger and Aggression 214
- Shadowing 224
- Sundown Syndrome 231
- Wandering 241
- Driving 254
- Refusing to Take Medication 260

Afterword 268
Dementia Resources 271
About the Author 273

Preface

If you're a dementia caregiver, take a moment to acknowledge and embrace the fact that you are an amazing person. Even under the worst circumstances, you're providing the best care possible for your loved one — whether they're living in your home or a care community. Your love and compassion are everlasting wherever they may be living.

Every day, I'm moved and touched by caregivers' inner strength. Your outpouring of compassion is a testament to your love, commitment, and dedication. This is especially true because the caregiver's journey can be difficult.

Caregivers share with me the guilt they feel for losing their temper when their loved one asks the same question for the thousandth time. They confess embarrassment about their desire to run away when their loved one follows them everywhere. They tell me they feel like a horrible person because they raise their voice when their loved one doesn't cooperate.

Your feelings and emotions don't negate the fact that you are an *amazing* person.

I'm dedicated to helping family caregivers navigate the dementia journey. I'm committed to providing caregivers with emotional support. I'm passionate about providing caregiver strategies designed to help diffuse challenging situations.

When I'm meeting with a client, I often end our conversation by saying, "Dementia has robbed you and your loved one of enough. *Please* don't let dementia rob you of your love, value, self-esteem, self-confidence, importance, and purpose!"

I'm sharing this message with all of the dementia caregivers around the world. I want to thank you for your love, care, and support on behalf of your loved one.

You are a blessing and a gift to those who know you. I'm holding you in my heart as you move through your journey.

With gratitude,
Tami Anastasia, MA

Introduction

> *The more knowledgeable you become about the progression of dementia, the better equipped you are to deal with the cognitive, physical, and emotional changes resulting from the disease.*

Your motivation in caring for a loved one diagnosed with dementia is likely a heart filled with love and compassion, and a desire to provide the best possible care. While caregiving can undoubtedly be a rewarding endeavor, your journey can also involve enormous demands and overwhelming challenges.

The more knowledgeable you become about the progression of dementia, the better equipped you are to deal with the cognitive, physical, social, and emotional changes resulting from the disease. Increasing your understanding of dementia and how it affects both you and your loved one will help you:

- Anticipate and prepare for what lies ahead;
- Navigate behavioral and cognitive changes;
- Develop effective coping skills and strategies; and
- Decrease the toll that caregiver stress, burnout, and depression can have on you.

Throughout this book, the term dementia refers to various forms of nonreversible memory loss or cognitive impairment. The tools and techniques detailed apply to caregivers of individuals with any form of dementia.

Being the caregiver for someone with dementia can be a lengthy journey. This book aims to provide you with a roadmap by:

1. Educating you about the progression of dementia so that you are better prepared to deal with its demands and challenges;

2. Empowering you as a caregiver and instilling confidence in your decision-making process; and

3. Equipping you with techniques and strategies to make your experience as loving, compassionate, supportive, and meaningful as possible.

The first section of this book focuses on how dementia affects your loved one and provides you with strategies to deal with the cognitive, physical, emotional, and social changes resulting from dementia.

The second section focuses on how caring for a loved one with dementia affects you and provides suggestions designed to lessen the physical, mental, and emotional toll of long-term caregiving.

The third section of the book focuses on 11 challenging behaviors common to those living with dementia. Using the 4 D's of Dementia Care — detach, document, diffuse, and distract — will help you pinpoint potential causes and solutions that will make your day-to-day life more manageable.

When you're on the caregiver's journey, it can be helpful to understand the experiences of other caregivers and their loved ones. Throughout this book, you'll read the stories of fictional families. These stories reflect the experiences of various clients I've had the privilege of working with over the years and the strategies I've taught them to use. For the purposes of this book, I've streamlined their stories and changed their names.

The truth is that the caregiver's journey isn't straightforward, and solutions aren't always easy to figure out. You may relate to some of these fictional families and their stories, which in turn can provide you with insight into your situation.

PART I
Dementia Basics

Defining Dementia

Dementia is a syndrome — a group of symptoms that are related — not a specific disease. It is a general term for the progressive decline in cognitive abilities that interferes with daily life due to the brain's physical deterioration. Those cognitive abilities include language, thinking, memory, problem-solving, and executive functioning. There are more than 100 types of dementia, including:

Alzheimer's Disease: Alzheimer's is the most widely known form of dementia. It manifests as an irreversible degeneration of language, memory, spatial orientation, thinking, problem-solving, and executive function skills. The symptoms gradually worsen over time. Eventually, the person with Alzheimer's becomes completely dependent on others for their care. Alzheimer's affects the part of the brain that controls thoughts, memory, and language, and eventually leads to complete brain failure and death; in fact, it's the sixth leading cause of death in the U.S.

Vascular Dementia: The second most common form of dementia is vascular dementia. According to some studies, it may account for 20 percent of the total number of dementia cases. Vascular dementia is brain damage due to reduced blood supply to the brain. This can be caused by mini-strokes that cause bleeding in or damage to the brain. It may also occur when a stroke restricts blood flow to the brain. It's important to note that many people who have mini-strokes or strokes never develop dementia. The symptoms of vascular dementia vary depending on which region of the brain is affected.

Parkinson's Disease Dementia: Parkinson's disease is a neurological disorder that causes tremors, muscle stiffness, shuffling gait, stooped posture, flat affect, and difficulty walking. People may have problems initiating movement, balance, and coordination. Usually, the symptoms begin gradually and worsen over time. Parkinson's causes changes in the brain that affect mental functions such as memory, concentration, judgment, and the ability to follow a sequence of steps to complete a task. The hallmarks of Parkinson's disease dementia are slowness in thinking and reasoning. Not everyone who gets Parkinson's disease will develop Parkinson's disease dementia.

Lewy Body Dementia: Lewy body dementia is also referred to as cortical Lewy body disease or diffuse Lewy body disease. It is the third most common reason for dementia. However, it is frequently misdiagnosed or underdiagnosed. Lewy body symptoms are best described as a combination of Parkinson's and Alzheimer's symptoms. The stiffness and rigidity associated with Parkinson's are grouped with the cognitive decline associated with Alzheimer's. One of the significant identifying factors of Lewy body dementia is visual hallucinations. The hallucinations can also be in the form of sounds, smells, or touch.

Frontotemporal Dementia: Frontotemporal dementia (FTD) is also known as frontotemporal lobar degeneration (FTLD) or Pick's disease. When the brain's frontal or temporal lobes — the parts of the brain behind the forehead and ears — deteriorate, FTD can surface. It is a much less common form of dementia. Someone with FTD experiences problems with language, along with significant changes in personality and behavior. The temporal lobe affects our ability to understand language, and the frontal lobe affects cognition, emotion, and voluntary movement.

FTD differs from other types of dementia in two important ways. First, it doesn't usually affect a person's memory as severely as Alzheimer's, but it does affect how a person behaves. It also impacts their personality, language, and ability to function. Second, the average age of someone diagnosed with FTD is 60 years old, which is younger than the average age of someone diagnosed with Alzheimer's or other dementias. Some experts call FTD the "young person's disease."

Head Trauma Dementia: When someone suffers a severe impact to the head, the resulting traumatic brain injury (TBI) can lead to learning and memory impairment. Depending on the type of TBI, there can be an increased risk of developing dementia many years after the brain injury. Currently, there isn't a body of research that suggests a single mild traumatic brain injury increases dementia risk.

Wernicke-Korsakoff Syndrome: Someone who has a thiamine (vitamin B1) deficiency can suffer from Wernicke-Korsakoff syndrome, a form of dementia often related to alcohol abuse. Thiamine deficiency means that the brain's hypothalamus doesn't get the energy it needs. As a result, the person can have amnesia, short-term memory loss, and mental confusion. Wernicke-Korsakoff syndrome is extremely underdiagnosed and is often misdiagnosed.

DEMENTIA

Dementia is a syndrome – a group of symptoms that are related – not a specific disease. It is a general term for the progressive decline in cognitive abilities that interferes with daily life due to the brain's physical deterioration.

Alzheimer's Disease
The most common form of dementia, Alzheimer's manifests as an irreversible degeneration of language, memory, spatial orientation, thinking, problem-solving, and executive function skills.

Vascular Dementia
Vascular dementia results from brain damage caused by reduced blood supply to the brain, often from stroke. The symptoms vary depending on which region of the brain is affected.

Lewy Body Dementia
Lewy body symptoms are physical stiffness and rigidity combined with cognitive decline. Hallucinations are an identifying factor of Lewy body dementia.

Frontotemporal Dementia
FTD symptoms include problems with language, behavior, emotion, and voluntary movement. Unlike Alzheimer's, memory isn't as significantly impacted.

Parkinson's Disease Dementia
The hallmarks of Parkinson's disease dementia are slowness in thinking and reasoning. Not everyone who gets Parkinson's disease will develop Parkinson's disease dementia.

Head Trauma Dementia
Depending on the type of traumatic brain injury, there can be an increased risk of developing dementia many years after the injury.

Wernicke-Korsakoff Syndrome
Caused by thiamine deficiency often related to alcohol abuse, someone with Wernicke-Korsakoff can have amnesia, short-term memory loss, and confusion.

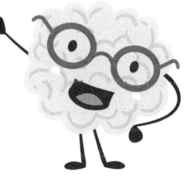

The Brain and Dementia

Our brains have billions of neurons. When someone has Alzheimer's, new neurons no longer generate. The result is called neurodegeneration. With neurodegeneration, the brain's neurons start to lose their structure, and brain cells die. As a result, the brain loses mass. This shrinkage of the brain is called atrophy. Atrophy occurs mainly in the hippocampus, the part of the brain that is responsible for memory and orientation.

Vascular dementia affects the brain's blood vessels, which transport the food and oxygen essential to normal brain functioning. When a stroke interrupts the brain's oxygen supply, neurons stop functioning properly or die in the part of the brain that is damaged. Vascular dementia can develop over time as the result of multiple strokes, though the symptoms depend upon the part of the brain damaged by the stroke.

Lewy body dementia is triggered when brain cells have protein deposits — called Lewy bodies — as well as plaques and tangles. These damage the neurons in various brain regions. The plaques and tangles also affect dopamine-producing neurons. Dopamine is a chemical substance that sends signals between two neurons and is needed for motor control, movement, and muscle coordination. If the Lewy bodies first form in cognitive regions of the brain, Lewy body dementia surfaces first. If the Lewy bodies first form in the areas of the brain that control motor function, then the motor symptoms of Parkinson's disease surface first. Eventually, those with Lewy body dementia experience motor control issues and those with Parkinson's may develop Parkinson's disease dementia.

How the Brain Changes During Alzheimer's Disease

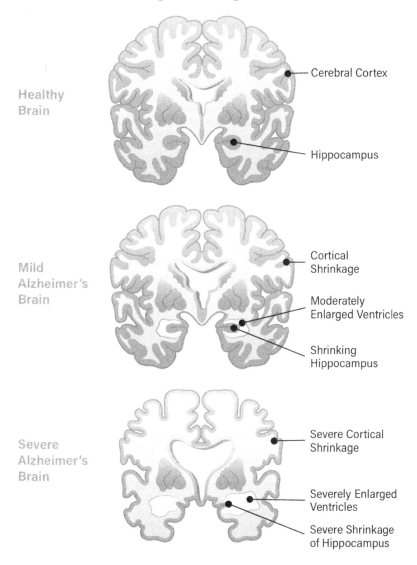

Over time, changes in the brain worsen the symptoms of Alzheimer's disease. Memory is affected when ventricles enlarge and the hippocampus shrinks. When the cerebral cortex begins to shrink, language, behavior, and bodily functions are impacted.

Regardless of the underlying cause of dementia, as the disease progresses, the brain cells lose their ability to communicate with one another, which causes brain damage. When the brain cells cannot communicate normally, a person starts thinking, feeling, and behaving differently. Eventually, when the neurons lose their ability to function correctly, the brain cannot survive. Total brain failure occurs, which results in death.

How Dementia Affects Your Loved One

Each family is unique. Each person with dementia and each caregiver is unique. Yet symptoms and challenges echo across families. As we delve into the various facets of dementia and how caregivers approach their loved ones, it's helpful to understand others' experiences. The fictional families described throughout this book provide snapshots of common caregiving scenarios. Their stories are based on real people, and the strategies outlined are those I've provided to caregivers and which they've put into practice. The purpose of telling these oversimplified stories is to let you know you're not alone, highlight possible solutions, and inspire you to keep trying. Our first family is Beth and Bob Brooks.

Beth and Bob married in their mid-20s. While Bob built a financial consulting business from the ground up, Beth raised their two children, Lucy and Lester, and was a valued volunteer at their local food bank. Thirty years into their marriage, Beth discovered that Bob was having a long-term affair. Although their marriage was on the rocks, the couple sought counseling and successfully weathered the storm. Recommitted to one another, the Brooks began dreaming of a European riverboat cruise to celebrate their 50th wedding anniversary. But it was not meant to be.

Shortly after Beth turned 70, Bob started to notice that his wife wasn't acting like herself. She was often forgetful, sometimes confused, and began misplacing everything from the car keys to her iPad. A visit with Beth's primary care provider led to an appointment with a neurologist, who conducted a battery of tests and brain scans. The diagnosis? Alzheimer's disease.

Over time, dementia affects Beth's ability to remember, think, speak, listen, process information, and care for herself. Like many people with dementia, Alzheimer's negatively impacts Beth's:

Short-term memory. People living with dementia don't remember things they said or did minutes or even seconds ago. Beth asks Bob when it's time for lunch — even though she's just eaten lunch. Throughout the afternoon, Beth asks dozens of times when their daughter is coming over, even though Bob has told Beth that Lucy is arriving at 6:00 p.m. It is common for people with dementia to repeat themselves. Doing so isn't an intentional effort to annoy you. They genuinely aren't aware that they've said the same thing 10, 20, or even 30 times.

Ability to think rationally and speak clearly. People living with dementia may say things and act in ways that don't make sense or aren't true. For example, when Beth can't locate her cash, she accuses Bob of stealing money out of her wallet. When she hides her keys in a tissue box and her purse in a bag in the far corner of a closet, Beth accuses Bob of taking her keys and purse. It's common for someone living with dementia to hide items in bizarre places and then accuse you of stealing, hiding, or losing their possessions. These interactions are known as "dementia accusations." It's how the person's brain makes sense of their world when they can't find items.

In your loved one's mind, there's no way they've misplaced something. The only explanation that makes sense is that you have taken it from them. Their brain creates an alternate version of reality. It's important to remember that they aren't saying or doing this to be hurtful. They have a brain disease that is causing them to do bizarre things, and their only possible explanation is that you must have moved the items they can't find.

Ability to process information logically. People with dementia eventually lose their ability to understand what is being said and won't be able to respond appropriately to normal conversation. As Beth's disease progresses, Bob realizes that he's no longer able to reason with her. Her ability to listen and logically process information has declined, and she is not able to have a rational conversation. This is because dementia affects the brain's ability to process and retrieve information.

Reading, writing, and communicating. Although Beth is a lifelong reader, Bob notices that she doesn't seem to be turning the pages in her book. Because of damage to some regions of the brain, your loved one may not understand what they have read, may have difficulty writing, and may not be able to find the right words when they are speaking. Eventually, they lose their ability to communicate clearly.

Recognition of familiar people, places, and things. As Beth's brain deteriorates, her memory loss becomes more severe. Familiar people, places, and objects become unfamiliar. Beth may lose her ability to recognize Lucy and Lester, or her own bedroom may become a strange place. People with dementia may forget their relationships with family and friends, call family members by the wrong names, or become confused about the location of their home or the passage of time. At some point, this may even include not knowing who you are.

Capacity for self-care. People living with dementia slowly lose their ability to perform daily activities, such as brushing their teeth, combing their hair, dressing, bathing, and toileting. As Beth's disease progresses, her ability to physically take care of herself declines. What once were considered simple tasks become very difficult for Beth to perform.

Ability to filter what she says. As Beth's brain deteriorates, dementia causes her to lose her ability to censor what she says. It is common for a person with dementia to blurt out inappropriate, offensive, rude, or embarrassing words. For example, Bob is flabbergasted when Beth uses a racial slur or makes a negative comment about her doctor's physical appearance.

Initiation and motivation. Dementia robs people of their ability to be self-starters. As time passes, Bob finds that Beth needs assistance starting projects and tasks. For example, he needs to set up and initially participate with Beth in putting together a jigsaw puzzle, folding napkins, and sweeping the floor. As a caregiver, you may need to simplify your loved one's tasks and activities according to their abilities. For example, you may need to buy puzzles with larger and fewer pieces that are easier to see and fit together. Or, you may need to set up and work with modeling clay until your loved one becomes occupied with the clay on their own.

Engagement with family and friends. As the disease progresses, people living with dementia tend to withdraw from family and friends. They can become introverts. For example, Beth resists leaving the house and loses interest in visiting with the neighbors. This occurs because dementia can cause anxiety, which leads the person to become increasingly fearful about leaving their home. Another reason people with dementia become withdrawn is because it is increasingly difficult for them to process information and engage in conversation. As a result, they can become overstimulated and overwhelmed, resulting in feelings of anxiety and frustration.

Ability to live in the present. The part of the brain that is most commonly affected by dementia is short-term memory. As the disease progresses, long-term memory is affected. As a result, people with dementia may not remember what they ate for lunch a few minutes previously but can remember events that occurred 20, 30, or 40 years ago.

Stages of Dementia

Here is a summary of what to expect during each stage of dementia:

Stage 1: Early (Mild Dementia)

You may notice subtle changes in your loved one's behaviors, thinking, and reasoning. They may be more forgetful, have trouble finding the right words, or demonstrate increased confusion with everyday tasks such as paying bills or cooking. They may misplace valuable objects. They may insist that nothing is wrong with them if these issues are pointed out to them. However, they're still able to maintain a certain level of independence by, for example, working, driving, and participating in social activities.

Stage 2: Middle (Moderate Dementia)

Your loved one's care needs increase significantly. For example, they may need more help with activities of daily living and may become more dependent on you to help them express themselves and perform routine tasks. They may need help with what clothing to wear and have trouble controlling their bladder and bowels. Typically, their sleep patterns change. They may have difficulty remembering personal history or be confused about events or where they are. They may become moody, withdrawn, or paranoid. This is also around the time concerns about their driving skills surface.

Stage 3: Late (Severe Dementia)

There is a dramatic decline in your loved one's cognition, mobility, and physical health. Their ability to communicate verbally and process information is impaired. They have difficulty swallowing, have urinary and bowel incontinence, and are more susceptible to infections. They may experience delusions and hallucinations, mood swings, and confuse the past with the present. At this point, 24-hour care may be critical for their safety.

Stage 4: End-Stage Dementia

Your loved one becomes incapacitated and is bedridden. They lose their appetite and are unable to speak, drink, or swallow. Support is needed to perform every function of daily living. The focus is on preserving your loved one's dignity and quality of life.

What Your Loved One Needs from You

As dementia progresses, your loved one's abilities decrease and their needs increase. As their needs increase, your role as their caregiver becomes increasingly demanding. Your loved one grows increasingly dependent on you for:

Reassurance and support. Someone with dementia needs reassurance that they're going to be okay and that their worry has been resolved. As their brain deteriorates, your loved one may bring up irrational concerns or fears that resurface from the past. For example, Bob is frustrated with Beth because she repeatedly accuses him of being unfaithful — even though he terminated his affair and the couple participated in counseling more than 20 years ago. But Beth's dementia makes her fear both real and immediate. She constantly needs Bob to provide comforting and reassuring responses to her accusations.

People with dementia need you to acknowledge their reality — even if it never occurred, happened in the past, or sounds ridiculous. Your loved one needs constant reassurance that you have the situation under control and that everything is fine. Your reassurance reduces their anxiety and comforts them — even if it's only temporary.

A sense of safety and security. As their dementia progresses, your loved one loses their ability to recognize familiar people, places, and objects. As confusion increases, your loved one becomes very concerned about their safety — where they live, who is taking care of them, and where they're going. Beth becomes dependent on Bob to make her feel safe and secure in their own home, when visiting with family and friends, and when going to medical appointments. She asks Bob where she is living. Bob responds by saying, "You're living in the house where we raised our children," and talks about fond memories they shared while living in that house. The more confused a person with dementia becomes, the greater their need to feel physically safe and secure — even if they have lived in the same home for 40 years.

Physical comfort and care. Eventually, people with dementia cannot care for themselves and lose their ability to communicate what they need. At that point, they may need assistance with brushing their teeth, grooming, dressing, toileting, and bathing. For example, as the disease progresses, your loved one's brain loses its ability to signal when they have to go to the bathroom. As a result, they have accidents. The person with dementia becomes unaware that they have soiled themselves and depends on you to keep them clean.

In addition, your loved one may be unable to communicate when they are in pain yet depend on you to ensure that pain is managed with medication. For example, Beth has a history of back problems, and Bob notices that she's pacing up and down the hallway. She refuses to sit down, saying, "It hurts." Bob decides to give her pain medication. After 15 minutes, she stops pacing and is willing to sit down in her favorite recliner.

If your loved one has dental issues, they may not be able to communicate that chewing food hurts; the only clue you may have is that they don't want to eat. They become dependent on you to figure out what is wrong and take them to the dentist. As the brain deteriorates, people living with dementia increasingly rely on you to care for their physical needs.

Validation. There is an innate need within each of us to feel heard and understood. This need becomes even more critical for those living with dementia. For Bob and Beth, this involves Bob acknowledging

Beth's concerns by listening and repeating back to Beth what she is telling him, even if he's heard it a million times, or even if what she's telling him doesn't make sense, isn't true, or is unrealistic. Validation involves listening, acknowledging, and repeating back word-for-word Beth's concerns, thoughts, and feelings rather than arguing, correcting, and challenging her.

Validation provides comfort and reassurance as your loved one becomes more confused, fearful, paranoid, anxious, or uncertain. Validation is a critical component of effective communication and makes the person with dementia feel heard. It's also a very effective way to diffuse challenging situations. For example, when Beth refuses to take her medication because she thinks it's poison, Bob doesn't argue with her. Instead of trying to convince her that the pill isn't poison, Bob instead acknowledges Beth's fear and doesn't force her to take her medication. Validating Beth's fear makes her feel safe and gives her a sense of control. Validation becomes increasingly important as dementia progresses.

Stimulation. Keeping your loved one's brain and body active is key to maintaining their quality of life. Yet, as dementia progresses, the person loses their ability to initiate and engage in cognitively and physically stimulating activities. In other words, they become increasingly dependent on you to provide the activities and encourage their participation in a variety of pursuits.

It's important to note that you must adapt activities to meet your loved one's cognitive and physical abilities. Activities must also align with their current strengths, abilities, and interests. If the activities are too advanced, your loved one may get frustrated and not want to participate. For example, during the early stage of dementia, Beth continued to enjoy constructing 500-piece jigsaw puzzles. As her disease progresses, she becomes frustrated and gives up. When Bob starts buying puzzles with fewer and larger pieces and helps her get started by separating the corners and edges, Beth once again becomes engaged in putting together puzzles.

A sense of purpose and value. Even as dementia slowly robs your loved one of their abilities, they still have a profound need to feel important and valued. Throughout Beth's life, she has had an identity. She's been a wife, a mother, and a valued food bank volunteer. That core person is still inside of her; it's Beth's brain that has become faulty. As her dementia progresses, Beth still needs to engage in ways that make her feel important, give her a sense of accomplishment, and provide her with a sense of purpose. She increasingly depends upon Bob to provide ways for her to feel useful and productive. He does his best to invite Beth to do tasks that match her physical and cognitive abilities, such as helping him with chores, accompanying him to the grocery store, or assisting him in solving a word search puzzle. Giving your loved one a sense of purpose requires engaging them cognitively, physically, and socially.

Your loved one also feels valued when you compliment them. For example, when you tell your loved one that they did a great job, that you appreciate them, or that you enjoy doing activities with them, it makes them feel special. Demonstrating affection also gives them a sense of belonging. Holding hands, a kiss on the forehead, or a hug conveys that they're important to you. This need doesn't go away because they have dementia; it lasts a lifetime. Your loved one may have a brain disease, but their soul needs to have a sense of purpose and they need to feel valued.

As the disease progresses, dementia incrementally robs your loved one of all of their abilities. Eventually, they need 24-hour care. Ultimately, you become the person who makes all of the decisions: medical, financial, legal, living arrangements, and end-of-life care.

Action Plan: Knowledge is Power

1. Has your loved one been diagnosed with a specific form of dementia? If so, which one?
2. Which symptoms of dementia is your loved one currently experiencing?
3. Based on your observations, what are your loved one's needs at this stage of the disease? Are they most in need of reassurance, stimulation, comfort and care, or something else?

PART II
Surviving the Caregiver Journey: PACE Yourself

Caring for a loved one with dementia involves dealing with a series of challenges. As dementia runs its course, your loved one's needs are in a state of constant flux. It is a laborious disease that takes a toll on both of you.

Your ultimate challenge and goal are to survive this journey while maintaining your physical, mental, and emotional well-being. This involves learning to PACE yourself.

PACE is an acronym, but it is also a roadmap:

P = Permission for Trial and Error
A = Acknowledge Their Reality
C = Compassionate Care
E = Empower Yourself

The PACE approach is essential throughout your journey because it enables you to:

- Conserve your energy;
- Make sure that your needs are met; and
- Acknowledge and accept your limitations.

Regardless of where you are on the caregiver journey, think of PACE as a toolkit. It is a framework to help you navigate the demands and challenges of dementia. Within these pages are insights, strategies, and explanations designed to make this journey easier on you. Whether you're feeling sad, frustrated, overwhelmed, or burned out, the PACE approach increases your self-confidence and provides you with valuable information that enhances your ability to make appropriate decisions. It helps you realize that you're not alone and that you're doing the best you can to care for your loved one.

PACE
P = Permission for Trial and Error

> **P = Permission for Trial and Error**
> A = Acknowledge Their Reality
> C = Compassionate Care
> E = Empower Yourself

Kathy and Jim are in their mid-50s and have three adult children and four grandchildren. Kathy's mom died of pancreatic cancer ten years ago. When Kenneth, her 82-year-old father, was diagnosed with dementia, he was initially able to live independently. As the disease progressed, though, Kenneth's ability to care for himself diminished. Kathy and Jim wrestled with whether to move him to assisted living or move him into their home. Ultimately, Kathy decided to take early retirement from her job as an analyst for the state to care for her father in the couple's home.

Throughout your caregiver journey, there are times when caring for your loved one is incredibly frustrating. Kathy's father, Kenneth, sometimes refuses her help. When Kathy places a towel on his chest to prevent him from spilling food on his clothes, he takes the towel off and sets it on the table. When she follows Kenneth to his bedroom to make sure he takes his shoes off before climbing into bed, he insists on leaving them on. In a role reversal from Kathy's childhood years, Kathy raises her voice and insists that her father cooperate. He reacts by pushing her away and telling her that he doesn't need her help. Kenneth tells her to stop treating him like a child and that he wishes she would leave him alone.

Invariably, Kathy gets frustrated and angry that her father rejects her help, and she resents that he makes more work for her. "If only he would cooperate and let me do things for him," she says to her husband, Jim. She is beside herself and exhausted.

Like Kathy, you may feel frustrated, angry, and completely worn out. The truth is, each person feels and expresses frustration differently. If you're holding down a job and caregiving, it may become increasingly challenging to juggle work and caregiving responsibilities. If you have school-aged children, you might feel like you're drowning or that you're spread too thin. There may be times when you are short-tempered and feel guilty about how you interact with your kids and with your loved one with dementia. Some caregivers become frustrated and angry at themselves for not being able to manage their responsibilities better. They may take those frustrations out on themselves, their loved ones, or their coworkers. The more frustrated a caregiver becomes, the more out of control they feel, and the more they blame themselves for not being a good parent, spouse, or child. Eventually, frustrations and anger take a toll, leading to caregiver stress and burnout.

The truth is, there isn't a one-size-fits-all solution to the challenges associated with dementia or those related to being a caregiver. What works for one person may not work for another. That's why it's essential to give yourself permission for trial and error. The point is to try a solution. If that strategy doesn't work, try another one. If that doesn't work, attempt a third. Don't expect yourself to be perfect; instead, give yourself permission to experiment. Sometimes, you figure out what works best by learning what doesn't work. While attempting and discarding specific strategies can be discouraging, give yourself time to figure it out. The key to this trial-and-error process is developing patience.

Developing Patience

When taking care of a loved one with dementia, you need to be prepared to go the distance. It's critical to conserve your energy so that when you get to the end of the dementia journey, it's not at the expense of your physical, mental, and emotional well-being. The more patience you develop, the less frustrated you are with your loved one and yourself. This preserves your precious energy. The goal isn't for you to be perfect. The goal is to reduce the frequency and intensity of your frustration so that it doesn't have long-term consequences for your health. The startling truth is that many caregivers pass away before their loved ones. Researchers at the University of Pennsylvania found that elderly caregivers face a 63 percent higher mortality risk than non-caregivers in the same age group. When researchers at Stanford University looked at Alzheimer's patients and caregiver mortality, they found that four in ten caregivers pass away from conditions related to stress before their loved one dies. The goal is to prevent this from happening to you.

Patience is a learned skill. It's not something that comes naturally, especially when you're in the throes of caring for a loved one living with dementia. But it does become a necessity when you're dealing with the unpredictable physical, behavioral, cognitive, and social changes that occur as dementia progresses.

The first step in developing patience is recognizing the warning signs of frustration and anger. Consider if and under what circumstances you:

- Are easily irritated;
- Become angry;
- Jump to conclusions;
- Raise your voice;
- Lose your temper;
- Feel overwhelmed;
- Cry;
- Feel hopeless;
- Lash out;
- Experience anxiety;
- Get headaches;
- Have digestive issues;
- Increase alcohol consumption;
- Feel guilty;
- Say things you regret;
- Are continually annoyed; or
- Feel resentful.

The second step in developing patience is to remind yourself that dementia is responsible for what your loved one says and does. Dementia — the disease, not the person with the disease — often places you in the undesirable position of having to make difficult choices and decisions. When you tell yourself that the disease is at fault, you're less likely to take your frustrations out on yourself or your loved one.

The third step is a natural outgrowth of the second: detach and try not to take what your loved one says and does personally. This is much easier said than done, but the more you make a conscious effort to remind yourself that dementia is responsible for the changes in your loved one, the more you are able to detach. To help you with this process, repeat to yourself several times each day, "The disease is causing my loved one to behave this way. The disease is causing my loved one to behave this way. The disease is causing my loved one to behave this way." Think of this as your dementia mantra. When you repeat this to yourself, eventually, your mind will shift gears and you'll become less reactive and more reflective.

The more you repeat this mantra, the more you are reminding yourself that you are not at fault and your loved one is not at fault for what you are both going through. It reinforces that the disease is what causes both of you to react and behave in specific ways. Learning to detach helps conserve your energy and allows you to develop effective responses and compassionate ways to approach your loved one.

Going back to our fictional family, Kathy is having difficulty accepting her father's limitations, and she's taking his rejection personally. She feels that Kenneth is intentionally being difficult and isn't considering the extra work he is causing. Kathy reminds herself that dementia is causing her father to behave in ways that create more work for her, and this awareness allows Kathy to step back and change how she interacts with her father.

Kathy's newly developed patience allows her to be reflective rather than reactive. For example, when she cooks Kenneth's favorite meatloaf, and he says that he doesn't like it, she doesn't take it personally and doesn't get angry. Instead, she detaches and reminds herself that dementia has changed her father's taste buds. Then, she finds a solution to the problem — she makes him a grilled cheese sandwich. In addition, Kathy develops a solid backup plan for when she gets angry: she walks away, goes into the bathroom to collect herself, and then comes back out when her patience returns.

The fourth step in developing patience is learning to refrain from internalizing your frustrations and blaming yourself or your loved one for what's happening. Kathy starts this process by reflecting on and thinking about the times Kenneth refuses her help and then looks for common denominators. She discovers that the common denominator is trying to force her father to do things on her terms to prevent more work for her. In reality, her father picks up on Kathy's assertiveness and her need to control the situation, and he fights back. Ironically, the more Kathy tries to exert control, the more frustrated she and her father become, but for different reasons. Ultimately, Kathy realizes that her father is not only reacting to her constraints but also her tone of voice, facial expressions, and lack of patience.

The fifth step in developing patience is identifying triggers and figuring out ways to respond in those situations. You have a long history with the person you're taking care of, and they may unintentionally say and do things that push your buttons. Your immediate response is to react defensively, which in turn makes things worse for you and your loved one. Understanding your triggers allows you to prepare responses in advance that are neutral rather than argumentative or confrontational. For example, when Kenneth accuses Kathy's husband of stealing Kenneth's money, she is initially furious, hurt, and outraged. Aware that her father has pushed one of her buttons, Kathy takes a deep breath and repeats the dementia mantra: "The disease is causing my loved one to behave this way." The mantra reminds her that dementia is responsible for her father's thinking and that he doesn't intend to hurt her with his accusations.

Rather than react angrily, Kathy steps back and asks herself, "How do I calmly respond to Dad's false accusation?" Instead of raising her voice and telling her father how insulting and absurd his accusation is, Kathy counts to three and uses one of her prepared responses. She says, "I'm sorry you can't find your money. I know where it is, and I'll bring it to you." Rather than react, Kathy acknowledges her father's frustration and provides a solution.

Kathy uses a similar approach when Kenneth repeatedly asks the same question. His constant questioning gets on her nerves and makes her want to pull her hair out. In the past, Kathy typically reacted by reminding her father that she had answered his questions a million times. The reality is that her father doesn't have control over asking the same questions, and Kathy needs to find a way to cope that conserves her energy. She decides to write down all of the questions that her father asks repeatedly. To her surprise, she learns that there are themes to his questions. He often asks when he will have his next meal, and he repeatedly asks what Kathy is doing that day. She comes up with two standard answers: "We'll eat soon," and "Today I'm doing housework and later we're going to spend time together." Once Kathy develops her go-to answers, she spends less time engaging in an endless back-and-forth exchange. She says these phrases and moves on.

The process of developing patience can provide you with insight, a sense of calm, and a feeling of being centered. When practicing patience, learn to take timeouts, count to three, and pause to take a deep breath. Deep, slow breathing is soothing, helps you become focused, and enables you to move forward with compassion and loving intentions.

At all times, remember that you're doing the best that you can. The best care you can give is doing what is best for you and your loved one. It's not one-size-fits-all. Often, the way to figure out what works best is by learning from what doesn't work. Mistakes are not failures — they are opportunities to learn.

Providing Structure

Example of a Daily Schedule	
8:30	Get out of bed; teeth, face, clothes
9:30	Breakfast and newspaper
10:30	Walk dog
11:00	Take bath or shower
12:00	Lunch
12:30	Music, mail, puzzles, games, or reading
1:30	Gardening, or call or visit friend
2:30	Exercise video
3:30	Backyard break
4:30	Help with chores
5:30	Help with dinner prep
6:00	Dinner
7:00	Play cards or game, or watch movie
9:00	Get ready for bed, read, listen to music
10:00	Bed

We often take for granted the stability provided by a consistent routine. Consider the transition that people go through when they retire. They were on a schedule throughout their school years, and then again for the 40 or 50 years spent in the workforce. With retirement, that schedule melts away, and they suddenly have an abundance of unstructured free time. Those in retirement often say that they don't know what to do with themselves, feel lost, or something is missing. This feeling is exponentially magnified for people living with dementia. Retirement can be difficult for those who don't know how to adjust to the lack of routine. For someone living with dementia, a lack of structure can cause anxiety, restlessness, agitation, and increased confusion.

Kathy took early retirement to care for her father, Kenneth. Initially, Kathy feels unsettled, unsure of how to go about life without the structure of her workday. As a new caregiver, she decides to follow her father's lead and tries to meet his needs as they come up. She quickly becomes frustrated because it seems that, as soon as she turns her back, he follows her around the house. He acts as uneasy as Kathy feels, repeatedly asking questions about what they will do today, when lunch will be ready, when they're going to the store, and when her husband will be home from work. Kathy resents not being able to get a moment to herself.

Kathy learns that people living with dementia need structure and that a visual schedule can be helpful. She buys a whiteboard and writes down the date, day, and time, and then lists their activities for the day. Kenneth can see the schedule from where he sits in his favorite recliner. She notices that her father starts to settle down, giving her room to breathe.

Creating a schedule for your loved one involves trial and error. It's essential to perform activities in the same order and around the same time every day. Studies have demonstrated that having a consistent routine decreases anxiety and improves sleep for those with dementia. Structure also provides your loved one with stability, predictability, normalcy, and a sense of purpose. Having a consistent routine makes them feel safe and secure. Importantly, it frees up your mental energy, allows you to have breaks, and gives you the time and space to do things you would like to do.

The importance of providing a schedule may seem counterintuitive when talking about those with memory impairments. However, just as people have muscle memory, everyone has body memory. Our bodies and minds have innate needs; maintaining a consistent routine is one of them. This doesn't go away just because your loved one has dementia.

As your loved one loses control over their physical abilities, cognitive functioning, and independence, they become increasingly confused and fearful. Structured, predictable days decrease their anxiety and stress. A consistent schedule provides a degree of normalcy for a disease that causes uncertainty.

Through creating and implementing a daily routine based on Kenneth's pre-dementia daily activities, Kathy finds that his level of cooperation increases and his adjustment to living in her home is smoother. For example, Kenneth always brushed his teeth, washed his face, and dressed before breakfast, so Kathy followed that schedule. Even though her father isn't consciously aware of the routine or realizes the passing of time, the schedule is familiar and he's less anxious throughout the day.

Action Plan: Nurturing Your Patience

1. List five habits you can implement that will help you build patience. It takes several weeks for an action to become a habit and even longer for that habit to become automatic. To begin, work on implementing the first strategy on your list. When that becomes second nature — whether in two weeks or a month — move on to the second strategy.

2. Routine is important. Create a daily schedule on whiteboards, easel pads, or large calendars. Post them where your loved one will frequently see them, such as near the front or back door, the kitchen counter, and on the wall near their favorite chair.

PACE
A = Acknowledge Their Reality

> P = Permission for Trial and Error
> **A = Acknowledge Their Reality**
> C = Compassionate Care
> E = Empower Yourself

Patricia and Peter were high school sweethearts, but then Patricia headed off to college in Los Angeles while Peter went to a New York university on an athletic scholarship. After going their separate ways, each eventually found love, married, and had a family. Patricia ultimately divorced her husband, while Peter's wife died in a car accident. While in their 50s, Patricia and Peter reconnected on social media. They rekindled their romance and married. A decade later, Peter got the devastating diagnosis of dementia, and Patricia embarked on the challenging road of caregiving.

Understanding Their World

> " Peace is the result of retraining your mind to process life as it is, rather than as you think it should be.
> — Wayne W. Dyer

Your loved one changes as their dementia progresses; as this happens, you may feel distant and disconnected. One of the biggest challenges is figuring out how to continue to connect and communicate with them as they drift away. The best approach is to meet them where they are. This means acknowledging their reality — especially when their reality doesn't match your own.

Understanding the communication challenges that dementia causes helps bridge the gap between their world and yours. These changes include:

- Short-term memory loss: They forget what is said or done within seconds or minutes.

- Increased confusion: They have difficulty following directions, have no sense of time, and confuse the present with the past.

- Inability to reason and process information logically: You can't reason with them.

- Repetitive thoughts: They ask the same questions again and again.

- Lack of awareness of limitations and deficits: They aren't aware that they repeat the same questions, hide items, or forget what you've told them.

- Rumination or fixation: They get stuck in looping or obsessive thinking.

- Basic expression: They have difficulty reading, writing, and speaking about their needs.

- Inability to filter what they say and do: They lack impulse control and act out or blurt out whatever they are thinking.

- Paranoia and accusations: They blame you or others for stealing or hiding items that go missing.

- Argumentativeness: They get defensive when you try to correct them because they believe what their mind tells them.

- Combativeness: They react defensively (e.g., hit, scream, kick, throw things, lash out, spit, pull hair, resist, refuse) when they feel threatened because they don't understand what you're doing.

- Confusing the past with the present: They may relive memories as though they are occurring in the present day.

While it's impossible to truly understand what your loved one is going through, it's easier to maintain your connection when you try to put yourself in their shoes. In doing so, you have a better understanding of how their brain is malfunctioning, which in turn helps you accept their altered version of reality — a reality that no longer coincides with yours.

For example, when Peter asks Patricia if she's ever met his wife, Patricia's heart drops. At that moment, Peter doesn't recognize that she is his wife. Patricia's participation in her caregiver support group has prepared her for this eventuality. She knows that it's best to meet Peter in his reality rather than to correct him. As a result, she encourages him to share more about his wife and asks him questions about what she's like and what he loves most about her.

By mirroring your loved one's experience, you communicate with them at their cognitive level. In other words, you meet your loved one where they are.

Acknowledging your loved one's reality is a key strategy in combating caregiver frustration. When your loved one says and does things that don't make sense, before you react or respond, ask yourself:

- How would you like someone to respond to you if you said or did the same thing?
- What tone of voice would you like to hear?
- What would you like the person's facial expressions and body language to communicate?

You would most likely want the other person to take what you say seriously and treat you with respect. In other words, you would like them to make you feel "normal." Given the circumstances, "normal" is relative, but you wouldn't want the other person to make you feel embarrassed, foolish, or stupid.

Taking it a step further, imagine if nothing made sense anymore. Imagine what it would feel like if everything that was once familiar is now unfamiliar: unfamiliar surroundings, unfamiliar people, and unfamiliar possessions. Picture how confusing, out of control, frightening, upsetting, and disturbing it would feel.

As a result of being confused and fearful, your loved one may say and do things that are bizarre, inappropriate, hurtful, or annoying. It's important to remember that their intention isn't to upset you. They say and do these things because they have a disease and, as a result, their brain isn't functioning correctly. For example, they may cling to you and follow you around because you become their security blanket. They may blame you for situations that aren't your fault. They may mistreat you or lash out at you because they don't understand what is happening around them. The only thing that makes sense to them is that you must be to blame for what's happening. As the disease progresses, they can't recognize or understand what is going on around them.

When Patricia helps Peter into the car, he shouts, "Who do you think you are? Don't treat me like I'm a prisoner! I'm an honest person. You don't have to check my pockets to see if I've stolen anything." Patricia is floored. Her instinct is to shout back at him. Instead, she says, "Of course you're not a prisoner. You're the most honest person I know, and you would never steal anything." Then, she immediately distracts him by asking Peter to tell her about the time he scored the winning touchdown in college.

Patricia's ability to step outside of the moment and generate a response that calms Peter down is the result of meeting her husband in his reality. This takes time, patience, and trial and error. Sometimes, Patricia is successful, and sometimes, her patience is worn thin and she reacts with anger. That's to be expected and is typical of the caregiver experience. You try, you stumble, and you try again. You do the best that you can.

As your loved one's brain deteriorates, they look to you to provide them with a constant sense of safety, stability, and reassurance. This involves understanding your loved one's new world, embracing them as they are, and being able to transition into their present moment.

Throughout Patricia and Peter's marriage, Thanksgiving was always the family's most important holiday. Peter always took center stage as he carved the turkey. They hosted festive Thanksgiving dinners for their children and grandchildren. As Peter's dementia progressed, Thanksgiving turned into a disaster. He could no longer carve the turkey, and the noisy family gathering overstimulated and disoriented him. With the help of her support group, Patricia allowed herself to mourn the loss of their traditional family get-together and understood the need to adapt to her husband's new world. The following year, her eldest daughter agreed to host the holiday meal. Patricia and Peter stopped by for a brief visit before returning home to a delicious, but subdued, Thanksgiving dinner. Patricia acknowledged her husband's fears throughout the day, reassured him, and did her best to make him feel safe and secure.

Understanding your loved one's inner life involves changing your expectations and embracing what is. It consists of letting go of what was and how you want things to be. It requires adapting to their new reality while living in your reality. It's learning to be flexible. Be patient with yourself as you try to juggle both worlds.

Reliving Past Trauma

> *A diseased brain relives past memories;*
> *a healthy brain represses past memories.*

Some people with dementia relive past experiences as though they are occurring in the present moment. Suppose your loved one experienced trauma, abandonment, or betrayal, or endured physical, psychological, emotional, or sexual abuse. In that case, they are highly likely to relive those experiences as though they're happening in the present moment. For example, Patricia is at her wit's end because she doesn't know what to do about Peter's irrational behavior. He's frantically packing two suitcases and wants to flee from the house.

Peter keeps yelling that it isn't safe to be here. "We need to leave before he gets home and hits us," he shouts.

It turns out that Peter's father was an alcoholic and would beat his children when he got home from the neighborhood bar. To escape his father's abuse, Peter would pack two suitcases, one for himself and one for his sister, and they would run down to the neighbor's house. Once Patricia realizes that Peter is reliving a past experience, she can console him and make him feel protected and secure.

When our brains are healthy, we can compartmentalize or repress traumatic memories, but as dementia progresses, memories or events can resurface. Different parts of the brain are responsible for various functions. Short-term memories are stored in the hippocampus, which is the area of the brain that is most affected by Alzheimer's disease. Long-term memories are stored outside of the hippocampus and therefore can remain intact longer. This is why people with dementia can recall or relive events that happened 30, 40, or 50 years ago but can't remember a conversation that occurred minutes ago.

Behaviors that appear odd or irrational may surface when reliving a past experience, whether that experience is traumatic or wonderful. Knowing your loved one's personal history and life experiences is tremendously valuable. The more you know about your loved one's past, the easier it is to comfort them when an old memory resurfaces.

Responding to Your Loved One

Each of us has an innate need — brain disease or no brain disease — to feel heard and understood. For those with dementia, feeling heard and understood provides comfort and reassurance. It's also the foundation upon which trust is built.

Acknowledging your loved one's thoughts, feelings, concerns, fears, and frustrations is particularly difficult when, at the same time, you're dealing with your feelings of loss, sadness, frustration, disappointment, and anger. As Peter's dementia progresses, Patricia's heartbreak increases. She mourns the years during their youth when they were thousands of miles apart, and she grieves the future that dementia robbed from them. As Patricia lies in bed at night, sorrow about the Hawaiian vacation they'll never take turns into anxiety about Peter's ongoing physical, emotional, cognitive, and social changes.

The emotional and cognitive changes caused by dementia can leave you wondering how to respond to your loved one's thoughts, feelings, and requests — especially when they're incorrect or unrealistic. When Peter tells Patricia that he has to finish a project at work, she knows that it's not true; he stopped working a few years ago. Still, she needs to acknowledge Peter's reality without triggering more of his anxiety.

You can acknowledge your loved one's reality in three steps: validate, empathize, and distract.

Step 1. Validate what your loved one says to you. Validation is one of the most effective ways of acknowledging your loved one. Validation is the act of repeating, paraphrasing, or reflecting to your loved one what they are saying. This is also known as reflective listening. When validating your loved one, use the exact words and language they use. For example, when Peter tells Patricia that he's concerned about a work project, she can respond by saying, "I know you are concerned about your work project." If he's angry that his daughter didn't call, Patricia can say, "I know you're upset that Samantha didn't call." Patricia is letting Peter know that she hears him and validates what he's saying.

When validating your loved one, keep it short and simple. Refrain from interrupting them, correcting them, giving them advice, or providing lengthy explanations. Those approaches increase agitation, frustration, and anger.

Two of the best phrases to use when validating people living with dementia are "thank you" and "I'm sorry." For example, you might say:

- "Thank you for sharing this with me."
- "Thank you for letting me know how you feel."
- "Thank you for bringing this to my attention."

Regardless of how upset they or you are, thank them for vocalizing their feelings and thoughts. Saying "thank you" diffuses, normalizes, and neutralizes whatever is on your loved one's mind.

Saying "I'm sorry" is an empathetic and validating response that conveys that you care and acknowledges how they are feeling. For example, you might say:

- "I'm sorry you feel embarrassed."
- "I'm sorry this is so hard on you."
- "I'm sorry that I upset you."

Apologizing serves to acknowledge and validate their feelings, enables you to take responsibility for causing distress, and diffuses potential outbursts or conflicts.

Other validating and comforting responses are:

- "Can you tell me more about that?"

- "I'll look into this for you."
- "I'll call them and find out."
- "I'll make sure to take care of it."
- "I can see how [upset, frustrated, angry, sad] you are."
- "I can see why you would feel this way."
- "I know how [upset, frustrated, angry, sad] this makes you feel."
- "I know you feel [dumb, frustrated]. Sometimes, I feel [dumb, frustrated] too when I…."
- "We'll get through this together."
- "I'd rather live with you than without you."
- "I'm thinking about you."
- "I love you."
- "I miss you."

Another good time to use validation is when your loved one requests something unrealistic. For example, when Peter tells Patricia that he wants to visit his deceased first wife, she can say, "Thank you for letting me know that you'd like to see Susan," instead of reminding him that she died many years ago. When Peter tells Patricia that he wants to go home — even though he's sitting in his living room — Patricia understands that, in Peter's reality, "home" is the house where he grew up. Patricia might say, "That is such a nice home," instead of telling him, "You are home."

Validating your loved one's requests acknowledges a need that they have. You may not always know what the need is — because it can vary from moment to moment and day to day — but it's crucial that you acknowledge what they are asking. They are trying to convey something of importance.

Empathetic Responses

> *Someone in the middle or late stages of dementia loses their sense of logic and ability to reason, and the truth may cause pain, distress, and mental anguish.*

Step 2. Answer your loved one's questions with empathy. Empathetic responses are reassuring and comforting, and they are essential when your loved one asks repetitive questions or is stuck on a specific topic.

Often, a person with dementia ruminates or fixates on a particular topic or question because they're expressing an underlying need. They may need reassurance, support, physical attention, cognitive stimulation, or a sense of purpose and belonging. It could be that they want to be the center of attention or share something important, or that they're concerned about an event or person.

While validation is an essential first step in empathy, the hard truth is that empathetic responses may involve withholding information or saying things that aren't entirely true.

Withholding information or embellishing the truth is a difficult concept for many people to accept. There is controversy surrounding which circumstance is worse: telling the person with dementia a lie to prevent emotional distress or telling them a truth that could cause emotional pain. Chances are, you were taught to never lie under any circumstances. As a result, your instinct is to be honest with your loved one. After all, telling the truth is the reasonable, moral, and ethical thing to do. However, when someone has dementia, you may need to make an exception to this rule. Someone in the middle or late stage of dementia loses their sense of logic and their ability to reason. Sometimes, the truth can cause emotional pain and mental anguish.

In dementia research, telling white lies or withholding information is referred to as therapeutic lying or compassionate fibbing. The intent behind therapeutic lying is to prevent people living with dementia from experiencing avoidable distress. When thought of in this light, a compassionate lie becomes a therapeutic act of kindness.

The purpose of withholding information or embellishing the truth is not to deceive the person with dementia; rather, it is to prevent them from getting upset, angry, or agitated. It's a way of joining their reality. Their brain cells are deteriorating, and they are living in a different world. Therapeutic acts of kindness acknowledge their reality by providing comfort and reassurance.

For example, after several years, Peter's dementia worsens to the extent that Patricia can no longer adequately care for him. She makes the heart-wrenching decision to move Peter into a memory care community. When she visits, Peter constantly asks, "When can I go home?" Patricia uses a therapeutic act of kindness when she says, "I don't know when you can go home, but I'll see what I can find out." Patricia's response acknowledges Peter's desire to go home and comforts him without making any promises.

Peter accepts Patricia's response because she's empathetically answering his question — even if she's not telling the truth. Because of his dementia, Peter has short-term memory loss and doesn't remember their conversations. When Patricia responds in the here and now, Peter feels validated and comforted knowing that she is looking into the situation.

In our world, you're telling your loved one a lie. But in your loved one's world, you are comforting them. The purpose of therapeutic acts of kindness is to spare people with dementia information that they may not understand or believe, or that could cause unnecessary emotional distress. It's a way to provide them with peace of mind — reassurance that they are safe and that their concerns are being addressed.

Depending on the severity of dementia, it is best to practice therapeutic acts of kindness when the truth could cause anguish, despair, anxiety, agitation, or confusion. When Peter asks how Susan, his deceased wife, is doing, Patricia simply says, "She's doing fine." Telling Peter that Susan is dead — forcing him to adhere to our reality — could be more detrimental than beneficial. She needs to allow Peter to live in his world, providing it's not hurting anyone.

Patricia learned about therapeutic acts of kindness the hard way. When Peter still lived at home, Patricia responded to the same question — "How is Susan doing?" — with the truth: Susan died decades earlier. Peter accused Patricia of lying to him. For several days, Peter was restless, agitated, and angry at her. He refused to talk to her, slammed doors, and tried to leave the house. With the help of her support group, Patricia realized that, rather than correcting, confronting, or explaining to Peter the reality of the situation, it's much better to acknowledge his need by validating it and giving him a comforting response.

Answering your loved one's questions using therapeutic acts of kindness is another way to meet them where they are. It's comforting, reassuring, and non-confrontational.

Using therapeutic acts of kindness is not meant to replace honesty if the person with dementia can accept objective reality. This ability varies from person to person. Some caregivers may never need to use therapeutic acts of kindness as a way of providing empathy. Validation and other empathetic responses may meet their needs.

There are other times when validation, putting yourself in their shoes, empathy, and therapeutic acts of kindness aren't enough to satisfy the person with dementia. During these times, you may need to redirect your loved one's attention by changing the topic or engaging them in activities they enjoy.

Distracting with Activities

As your loved one's cognitive abilities decline, they may become anxious, frustrated, confused, fearful, and paranoid. Sometimes, validation and empathy may not be enough to comfort them, especially if they are ruminating, obsessing, or repeating themselves. That's when the third step is necessary.

Step 3: Using activities to distract. The purpose of distraction is to redirect your loved one's attention. The method of distraction is to engage them in an activity. For example, when Peter ruminates about his non-existent work deadline, he gets agitated. Using trial and error, Patricia has learned to redirect his attention by bringing out a set of dominoes, asking him to help her complete a puzzle, or inviting him to dance with her.

Activity Ideas

There are many different types of activities that can be adapted to your loved one's interests and abilities, including:

Helping	Baking, drying dishes, dusting, sorting silverware, sweeping the patio, sorting coins, folding laundry, organizing cans in the pantry, stirring cookie batter
Games	Checkers, dominoes, jigsaw puzzles, rummy, Old Maid, tic-tac-toe
Art	Modeling clay, painting, drawing, crafts, coloring
Entertainment	Movies, sports games, music, looking at magazine photos, reading the newspaper, going out for a treat
Reminiscing	Old photos, favorite memories, family stories, favorite jokes
Gardening	Gardening: Planting flowers, watering plants, weeding flower beds, raking leaves
Movement	Walking, dancing, playing catch, chair exercises, exercise bands, light hand weights, stretching, tai chi, yoga, stationary bike, balance exercises
Small pleasures	Scenic drives, backyard bird watching, eating favorite foods, holiday traditions, singing songs, reading the newspaper, attending worship services
Problem-solving	Changing batteries in a flashlight, word search puzzles, tightening screws, rolling yarn, putting items in a box to fill

Generally speaking, activities for those with dementia can be broken down into five categories:

Helper Tasks: Someone with dementia experiences that all-important sense of purpose when helping. Examples of helper tasks are folding towels, washing dishes, cleaning the sink, sorting coins, counting plastic utensils, and sweeping the floor.

Problem-solving Activities: Successfully finding a solution reinforces confidence and instills a sense of accomplishment. Although some activities, such as word search or jigsaw puzzles, specifically tap into problem-solving abilities, virtually any activity can incorporate finding solutions. The idea is to start an activity together and have them complete it. For example, Patricia sometimes asks Peter to finish connecting the dots, fill in the missing X or O in a tic-tac-toe game, or switch out the batteries in their flashlight. If your loved one likes to sing, you can pretend to forget the words to a song and have them sing the words. If they're artistically creative, you can ask them to help complete a drawing you began.

Leisure Activities: Everyone — including people with dementia — enjoys relaxing and being entertained. Watching favorite movies, going for scenic drives, playing games, or eating favorite foods redirects your loved one's attention and provides pleasure.

Physical Movement: Your loved one is less anxious when their blood is circulating and their muscles and joints are moving. This isn't about meeting exercise goals — it's about moving their body. Peter joins Patricia in doing chair exercises, going on walks, and gardening. Perhaps you can encourage your loved one to walk up and down the hallway, follow along with a yoga video, play catch, garden, or play balloon volleyball.

Togetherness: Togetherness includes a broad range of activities that make the two of you feel connected. Patricia misses intimacy with Peter, so she demonstrates her affection by holding his hand, giving him a kiss, or putting her arm around his shoulders. You can reminisce with your loved one about the good old days, places you traveled, and people you met along the way. You can tell your loved one that spending time together makes you happy and that you enjoy being with them.

Complimenting your loved one and inviting them to participate in an activity can be an effective way of distracting and engaging them. The following phrasing is often helpful when using an activity to distract someone with dementia:

- "I love it when we spend time together. It would be so much fun if we could [activity] together now."
- "I'm so glad we're spending time together working on [activity]. It's more fun when we do this together."
- "Can you show me how this works? You're better at figuring things out."
- "You're such a great helper. Can you do [helper task]?"
- "You have such a great sense of humor. Can you tell me that funny story again?"
- "I love when you tell me stories — can you tell me about…"
- "I'm in the mood for ice cream. Let's get some ice cream before we do [activity]."

- "You do such a good job helping me with [helper task]. Can you help me with [new task]?"
- "When you do [activity], it's such a big help to me. Thank you!"
- "I don't like to do [activity] alone. Would you do it with me?"
- "Would you keep me company and help me work on [activity]?"

The point is to use phrasing that is complimentary and inviting. This gives your loved one a sense of purpose and a feeling of importance. Note the use of the word "we." Saying "we" invites cooperation and gives your loved one a sense of inclusion. It implies that the two of you are a team and are working together.

When you're using activities as a distraction, it's essential to choose those that your loved one likes to do and that match their ability level, which can vary from day to day. Start by writing down a list of a dozen activities that your loved one enjoys. Keep your list handy and, when they're agitated, invite them to engage in one of the activities on the list.

Remember to modify or simplify these activities according to your loved one's cognitive and physical abilities. When you engage them in activities that exceed their abilities, they can become frustrated or angry, which is the opposite of what you're trying to accomplish. For example, Peter has always enjoyed the short stories and quotes in *Reader's Digest* and is content when Patricia reads to him. Thinking she could engage him cognitively, Patricia asks Peter to read some passages to her. Peter angrily refuses and insists that Patricia put the magazine away. In truth, like many people with advancing dementia, Peter has lost his ability to comprehend what he reads, and being asked to read agitates him because it reinforces what he can no longer do.

It's important to note that these three steps — validate, empathize, distract — must occur in order and quick succession. First, validate what your loved one has said. Second, empathetically respond to them by providing a comforting response. Third, provide a distraction by changing the topic or getting them involved in an activity they enjoy. This three-step process is very effective because it takes their mind off the issue concerning them.

Because dementia causes short-term memory loss, your loved one is easily distracted. This serves you well when they are asking questions or making unrealistic requests. This three-step process also helps diffuse potentially challenging behaviors.

Here's an example of the three steps in action when the person with dementia says, "I want to go home."

Validate: "Thank you for letting me know that you would like to go home."

Empathize: "It's lunchtime right now, so let's eat lunch first."

Distract by Reminiscing: "I love when we have lunch together. It reminds me of the time you surprised me with a weekend in San Francisco. We ate lunch at Fisherman's Wharf, and the next day we went to a Giants' game."

Distract with an Activity: "I love when we have lunch together. Let's work on the puzzle we started."

As your loved one's brain cells deteriorate, your loved one becomes more confused, fearful, anxious, and uncertain about people, places, and things that were once familiar. As a result, they increasingly depend on you to make them feel safe and secure. Acknowledging their thoughts and feelings, providing empathetic and comforting responses, and redirecting their attention are compassionate and loving forms of communication.

Action Plan: Response Preparedness

1. Having prepared responses conserves your energy and enhances communication between you and your loved one. Write down three or four validating statements and three or four empathetic statements that you can say when your loved one is distressed or repetitive. Once those statements come second nature to you, you can expand your repertoire.

2. Make a list of six to eight activities that your loved one enjoys and that you can do quickly if you need to redirect their attention or distract them.

3. Fill a bin or drawer with supplies for activities. It might contain games, a deck of cards, art supplies, yarn, nuts and bolts, poker chips, old photos, nature books, or whatever your loved one enjoys. Having supplies in one place allows you to have distractions at your fingertips.

PACE
C = Compassionate Care

> P = Permission for Trial and Error
> A = Acknowledge Their Reality
> **C = Compassionate Care**
> E = Empower Yourself

Debra and DeShawn met in their late 30s, when they worked for the same law firm. Debra was a fierce litigator, a force to be reckoned with in the courtroom. DeShawn took the spotlight in mergers and acquisitions, ironing out thorny issues that arose during negotiations. When they married, their blended family of four children thrived. Now in their early 70s, Debra has Alzheimer's. Even though all but one of their adult children live in a 60-mile radius, DeShawn struggles to care for Debra.

Having the Conversation About Dementia Care Options

Primary caregivers have a tremendous amount of guilt and angst when it becomes necessary to provide additional care for their loved one. When it becomes clear that Debra needs more care than DeShawn can provide, he wants to make the decisions that honor his wife's wishes — but they never had that conversation. Like most couples, Debra and DeShawn talked about their future, but their plans and promises didn't factor in a dementia diagnosis.

One of the most important things you, your loved one, and your family can do after a dementia diagnosis is to educate yourselves about the progression of the disease and have realistic discussions about the care needed as dementia progresses. While most people wish to be cared for at home, this isn't always realistic, and primary caregivers are often forced to make difficult decisions.

It's ideal to discuss care options with your loved one and your family while the person with dementia can comprehend and articulate the long road ahead. It's best to have this discussion before they need help with activities of daily living; cognitive, physical, or social stimulation; or companion care. Start by becoming acquainted with the different dementia stages and accompanying symptoms. This allows everyone to openly discuss and prepare for your loved one's long-term care.

At some point, you cannot care for your loved one by yourself. The expectation to do so is both unrealistic and unfair to you. Eventually, your loved one's mobility will be affected, and they will need assistance with sitting, standing, walking, and transferring from one position to another. They will need help with personal hygiene and may refuse or forget how to bathe, toilet, or dress. Your loved one's safety will be jeopardized due to falling more frequently or wandering away from you or the house. It becomes challenging to prevent dehydration, urinary tract infections, vitamin D deficiency, and B12 deficiency. Your loved one may start acting out, becoming aggressive, combative, or agitated. It's crucial to enlist extra support.

The reality is that it takes more than one person to help manage the symptoms of advanced dementia. Discussing your loved one's future care options with them or your family helps reduce caregiver guilt, shame, and anxiety. Even if your loved one disagrees, is argumentative, or gets upset when you bring additional care into the home or move them into a care community, you will feel better knowing that you had this conversation ahead of time.

Topics for discussion after receiving a dementia diagnosis include:

Cognitive and social stimulation: Your loved one will need to participate in cognitive and social activities to keep their brain engaged and active. This will require additional resources. Discuss available options, such as hiring an activity specialist to come to the house, going to a senior daycare or activity center, or moving into a care community.

Companion care: Your loved one will need more one-on-one interaction. Discuss the various options available, such as family and friends who can take them on errands, come over for visits, play games, or take them out to eat. Another option is to hire a professional caregiver from a home care agency or place your loved one in a care community.

Personal hygiene and physical care: Your loved one will need assistance with physical movement and personal hygiene tasks, such as dressing, bathing, and toileting. These become very challenging to manage as the disease progresses. Talk about bringing in additional care and support, such as hiring in-home care or moving your loved one into a care community.

Driving: At some point, your loved one will need to stop driving. Figure out how to handle this situation, and ask your loved one to sign a document stating that they agree to give up driving when specific warning signs occur. Warning signs include:

- Getting lost going to familiar places;

- Poor decisions and judgment;
- Confusing the gas and brake pedals;
- Driving exceptionally slow or fast;
- Inability to stay in their lane;
- New dents or scratches on the car;
- Driving over curbs;
- Not obeying traffic signs and signals;
- Acting more agitated, impatient, or angry while driving; or
- Receiving complaints from friends and family about your loved one's driving.

If the time comes and they aren't willing to stop driving, then you need to consider other options. You may have to contact the motor vehicle department or ask their doctor to notify them. You might have to make the car inoperable, hide the car keys, have the vehicle towed, or ask a friend or relative to drive the car for them.

There are two primary goals in discussing these issues in advance. The first is to decrease the degree of guilt that you, as the primary caregiver, struggle with throughout the dementia journey. The second is to line up resources ahead of time so you're as prepared as possible when the time comes.

Before the disease progresses, encourage your loved one to give you permission to do what is necessary to provide them with the best care. This makes you feel less alone in the decision-making process.

Imagine if Debra and DeShawn had a conversation that went something like this:

What if Debra had said: "I know you will take excellent care of me. I want you to trust your decisions on my behalf because you will be making those decisions with my best interests at heart. I will slowly lose my ability to communicate this message to you and, no matter what happens — if my personality changes, or if I say and do hurtful things, or if I don't cooperate when you're trying to help me, or if I react combatively — I'm not doing this intentionally. It's dementia causing me to do these things. Every step of the way, know that I love you and thank you. I support whatever decisions you make, even if I don't express my support, and instead, I get angry or appear unhappy. Please know that my reactions aren't because you're making the wrong decisions. My reactions are because of dementia. I want to apologize in advance for what you may go through while taking care of me. My inability to express my gratitude will be due to dementia, but know that I am grateful for everything you do for me. This is true even if it means I need to be moved to a care community. Please remember my words and not what dementia takes away from me."

What if DeShawn had said: "I want you to know that I will do my best to provide you with the best quality of care. I will make decisions with your best interests at heart. I may not always know how to deal with challenging situations and behaviors, but I will figure it out. I will never intentionally hurt you or embarrass you. When things get difficult, my intention is not to make you angry or upset. I may not be able to care for you alone. If I need to bring in outside support, it's not because I'm giving up on you. It's because I need help providing you with the care and support you deserve. I will always treat you with respect and dignity. We're in this together —

even when you're afraid I'm going to leave you. I will do everything in my power to maintain your highest quality of life, and I will love you to the very end. Please know that my love, commitment, and devotion to you don't change because of dementia."

If you don't get the opportunity to discuss these issues with your loved one or with your family in advance, know that you are doing your best to provide your loved one with excellent care.

Communicating with Kindness

12 Keys to Compassionate Communication

1. Be aware of your body language, tone of voice, facial expressions, gestures, and posture.
2. Replace "you" with "we" and "us."
3. Keep questions and answers short and simple.
4. Simplify the decision-making process by giving your loved one only two choices.
5. Avoid asking, "Why?" and "Remember?"
6. Speak slowly.
7. Make eye contact.
8. Limit distractions, such as loud noises, TV, and several people talking all at once.
9. Avoid arguing, correcting, explaining, and rationalizing.
10. Walk away if you're frustrated or angry.
11. Avoid telling your loved one no, that they need help, or that they can't or shouldn't do something.
12. Focus on the things they can do rather than those they can't do.

As someone who doesn't have dementia, you can communicate your needs directly and clearly. In contrast, your loved one with dementia eventually loses the ability to communicate their needs clearly and becomes dependent upon you to take care of those needs. In addition, they lose their ability to process information and become sensitive to your tone of voice, facial expressions, and body language.

As Debra's disease progresses, DeShawn finds that communicating with her becomes increasingly challenging. Debra not only has more difficulty communicating her needs but also has difficulty processing what he says. DeShawn notices that his wife doesn't always comprehend what he's saying and that she sometimes has a blank look on her face or stares into space. It's not that Debra isn't listening or deliberately refuses to understand what DeShawn is saying; rather, it's that she can't process what he is saying. The vacant look and unfocused eyes are non-verbal cues that Debra is having difficulty following what her husband says to her.

There are several strategies you can use to address communication challenges.

Use comforting body language: According to the Alzheimer's Association, body language is 55 percent of communication, tone of voice is 38 percent, and only 7 percent is verbal. This means that the words you choose become less important over time, and your facial expressions, mannerisms, and tone of voice become more important to your loved one. They pay close attention to your body language as a way to make sense of the world around them. It's one way to compensate for what they can't process. If your loved one senses that you are impatient, upset, angry, or frustrated, they are likely to react negatively. If they sense that you are happy or cheerful, they are likely to remain calm.

Previously, when it was time to leave for a doctor's appointment, DeShawn raised his voice, threw his hands in the air, frowned, and said, "What is taking you so long?" As a result, Debra became anxious and lost track of what she needed to do before leaving. Realizing the effect of his behavior on her, DeShawn figures out that he needs to give Debra more time to get ready. As a result, he schedules medical appointments later in the day and starts the process of departing two hours earlier. This allows Debra time to go through her ritual of stacking napkins, finding her purse, and putting on her coat. Because DeShawn accommodates his wife's slower pace, he's calmer and more patient. Instead of getting exasperated and yelling at Debra, he smiles when she's ready and affectionately takes her hand once they get into the car. As a result, they arrive at Debra's appointments on time and without drama and upset.

Even though your loved one may not understand your words, your body language and tone of voice speak volumes. For example, sitting and smiling or speaking in a soft tone conveys calm reassurance. In contrast, placing your hands on your hips or speaking rapidly in a high-pitched tone communicates frustration and impatience. Do your best to be aware of your body language and speak in ways that take into consideration your loved one's limitations.

It's equally important to pay attention to your loved one's body language so that when they can't communicate their needs, you can figure out what their needs might be. For instance, pay attention to what their eyes are telling you, what their facial expressions mean, and what their tone of voice is conveying. This becomes extremely important as the disease progresses.

When DeShawn puts these compassionate communication strategies into practice, he better understands his wife's needs, and Debra processes information more easily.

Keep questions and explanations short and simple. Ask one question at a time. The fewer the number of words, the better. For example, when it's time for Debra to eat breakfast, DeShawn doesn't ask, "What would you like for breakfast?" Instead, he says, "It's time for us to eat breakfast. Do you want cereal or eggs?" Simplifying the decision-making process by using a gentle tone of voice, making a statement, and providing two choices has three benefits: it conserves your energy; it allows your loved one to process what you're asking; and it includes them in the decision-making process.

In contrast, asking open-ended questions or verbalizing your train of thought can be difficult for your loved one and exasperating for you. Debra is completely lost when DeShawn says, "I'm thinking of what to cook for dinner tonight. I can't decide whether to cook salmon and vegetables, hamburgers and fries, or soup and sandwiches. What do you prefer to eat for dinner tonight? What are you in the mood for?" This is too much information for Debra to process. The longer DeShawn talks, the more difficult it is for Debra to decide because she can't follow or process everything he says.

The goal is to simplify, simplify, simplify. The same holds true for explanations. For example, when it's time to take Debra to a doctor's appointment, DeShawn doesn't mention why they're going to the doctor. Instead, he says, "It's time to put our shoes on so we can go see Dr. Hodges." In contrast, DeShawn expends unnecessary energy and overwhelms Debra when he says, "We need to leave in 30 minutes to go see the doctor so he can check your heart and your blood pressure. The doctor wants to make sure the new medication is working. You need to get ready and put your shoes on, so we're not late. Do you know where your shoes are?" Simplify the communication process to make it less frustrating for both of you.

Avoid questioning or making demands of their memory. Assume your loved one isn't going to know why they did something or even remember that they did it. Avoid testing their memory by asking them, "Why?" or if they remember an event, person, or place. It's tempting to want answers, but questioning your loved one is not productive or beneficial for either of you. Stay away from these kinds of questions and statements:

- "I've told you this a million times, don't you remember?"
- "I'm getting tired of repeating myself. You need to try and remember the things I tell you."
- "You did that yesterday. Why are you doing it again?"
- "I've answered that question five times. Don't ask me again."
- "I've told you not to do that. Why are you doing that?"

Put yourself in their shoes. Think about how it might feel being on the receiving end of this line of questioning. In addition, asking your loved one why and if they remember can be perceived as intentionally mean or hurtful.

Don't argue, correct, explain, or rationalize. People living with dementia have a brain disease. The disease is killing healthy brain cells. Therefore, their brain isn't functioning properly. This means that your loved one says and does things that don't make sense, are incorrect, or may even be inappropriate or embarrassing.

When Debra tells DeShawn that she lives in Illinois — when, in fact, they live in California — DeShawn corrects her. As a result, Debra becomes angry and argumentative. DeShawn learns that Debra believes what her mind tells her and that correcting her isn't helpful. Instead, he steps into her reality and invites her to tell him more about living in Illinois. He asks Debra what she likes most about living in Illinois and how long she's lived there. Asking these questions provides DeShawn with the opportunity to collect more information about the time period in which Debra's brain exists. He discovers that Debra thinks she's at the University of Chicago, where she went to college. This gives him the timeframe in which Debra believes she's living and allows him to interact with her in her reality.

Arguing with your loved one, correcting them, explaining to them, and trying to be rational with them are counterproductive ways of communicating. In fact, challenging your loved one often frustrates and angers them because they genuinely believe what their brain is telling them. Confronting your loved one can also make them defensive, which can lead to mistrust and accusations. This can become a serious problem because dementia can cause paranoia. You don't want to reinforce the paranoia and distrust that can develop from dementia.

Speak slowly and clearly. It takes longer for people living with dementia to process what's being said, so give your loved one the time they need. When you have to repeat yourself, say the exact same thing in the same way. Slow down and enunciate your words. For example, when DeShawn says to Debra, "It's time for us to go to bed," and Debra doesn't respond, DeShawn repeats the same phrase and then starts the process of getting ready for bed. He doesn't go into a lengthy explanation of why it's time for bed and all of the steps involved in getting ready for bed. For Debra, repetition is comforting and reassuring while enabling DeShawn to achieve his desired result without becoming frustrated or exhausted.

Make eye contact. Peripheral vision decreases as dementia progresses. It's important to be at your loved one's eye level and within their peripheral vision when you're speaking. For instance, don't speak standing up if they're sitting down. Maintain eye contact and avoid becoming distracted.

Use short sentences. Long or complex sentences can be overwhelming for a person living with dementia because they cannot process that much information. At first, it can feel awkward to say less, use shorter sentences, and ask direct questions. In fact, you may feel as though you're abrupt and rude. In reality, saying less and speaking more directly is respectful of their limitations and makes your loved one's life easier.

Focus on what they can do. There is a tendency to focus on what people living with dementia can't do. When you tell them, "No," "You need help," "You can't," or "You shouldn't," they may become defensive. Instead, try to communicate in ways that focus on what they can do. For example, Debra wants to clear the dishes off the table and tries to carry all of the dishes at once. DeShawn knows this is both dangerous and impossible. Instead of telling her that she can't clear the table, DeShawn anticipates Debra's need. He preemptively starts collecting the dishes and gives her two dishes to carry. DeShawn kindly asks Debra if she can help him, making her feel useful. Or, he distracts Debra by asking her to turn on the water while he brings the dishes to the sink. The key is to divert her attention and communicate in ways that support what she can do. This involves taking the initiative and substituting what she can't do with something she can do.

Provide visual and verbal cues. As your loved one loses their ability to understand your words, providing visual cues can help them follow what you're saying. Showing, telling, and gesturing are especially helpful when you want your loved one to:

- Brush their teeth;
- Change clothes;
- Get dressed;
- Put on shoes;
- Drink from a glass or mug;
- Take a shower;
- Take medication;
- Follow you or move in a specific direction;
- Get up from a chair;
- Sweep the floor;
- Wipe the counter;
- Wash or dry the dishes;
- Dust the furniture;
- Sit on the toilet; or
- Sort or stack items.

If your loved one has a blank stare or dazed look on their face, they likely don't understand what you want them to do. Demonstrating the task while repeating your request can result in a more successful outcome.

> ❝ I've learned that people will forget what you said, people will forget what you did, but people will never forget how you made them feel.
> — Maya Angelou

Respond to feelings. As a caregiver, one of your biggest challenges is focusing on your loved one's feelings rather than their actions. Listening to feelings is different than taking what someone says at face value. You need to pay attention to their tone of voice, facial expressions, posture, body language, and the emotions behind their words.

For example, when Debra gets up from the table and says, "I hate jigsaw puzzles," DeShawn looks beyond her words and sees that she's frustrated. He responds by saying, "I'm sorry this is so frustrating for you. Sometimes, I feel the same way when I put together this puzzle. Let's go for a walk instead." Or, he might say, "This puzzle is difficult for me, too. Let's get a snack." The key is to try and identify the underlying emotions your loved one is expressing and immediately comfort them by validating their feelings and redirecting them to an activity they enjoy or that is easier for them to do.

Even if your loved one is accusatory, focus on the emotions they are expressing. For example, when Debra accuses DeShawn of hiding her purse, he responds by saying, "I know it makes you angry when you can't find what you're looking for." Or, he might say, "I'm sorry. I know it's upsetting when you can't find your purse."

Your loved one's disability causes cognitive impairment, memory loss, inability to process information, distorted thinking, and unpredictable emotions and behaviors. Not remembering, not understanding, constant repetition, not knowing "why," and saying things that are incorrect or don't make sense is normal behavior for people with dementia. Modifying how to communicate with your loved one is a significant way to conserve your energy. Essentially, it's a win-win for both of you.

> *One person caring about another represents life's most significant value.*
> — John Rohn

These strategies can help you maintain positive communication with your loved one:

- Try not to rationalize, argue, explain, challenge, or correct your loved one when they are wrong unless they're in an unsafe situation.
- Try not to convince them of your way of thinking.
- Try not to be invested in being right or proving a point.
- Try to avoid being forceful or insistent. Instead, be flexible and accommodating.
- Try to avoid becoming frustrated. Instead, focus on validating and being empathetic. Remind yourself that your loved one has a brain disease.

- Try to avoid asking open-ended questions or questions that require detailed answers.
- Try to avoid asking them why or if they did something.
- Try to avoid challenging their memory.
- Try not to ask them if they remember, and don't remind them if they forget.
- Try not to give detailed or lengthy explanations.
- Try not to take what your loved one says and does personally.

Remember, dementia is causing your loved one to have an altered state of reality. Changing how you communicate with them is essential in order to maintain your emotional, physical, and mental well-being.

In addition, changing how you communicate with your loved one allows you to meet them where they are and establish a meaningful relationship on their level. Even though they have dementia, you can still find ways to connect with them, but it requires letting go of what was and how you want them to be. Instead, accept what is and focus on what your loved one is still able to do.

Having Compassion for Yourself

Dementia is a disease that affects the entire family. Watching a loved one slowly decline especially impacts you as the primary caregiver.

Dementia is a disease that affects the entire family. Watching a loved one slowly decline especially impacts you as the primary caregiver. Throughout this journey, you may ask yourself:

- How do I deal with my conflicting feelings and emotions?
- How do I stay strong for my loved one when inside I want to scream or cry?
- How do I deal with feeling trapped and wanting to take time out for myself?
- How can I take care of myself when I'm exhausted from taking care of my loved one?
- How do I deal with the guilt of wanting to do things that my loved one can no longer do?

If you're like most dementia caregivers, you may feel conflicted between taking care of yourself and taking care of your loved one. It's often easier to put your life on hold and neglect your own needs.

Studies show that caregivers often neglect themselves when taking care of someone with dementia. They may suffer in silence or feel guilty when they can't meet the demands and responsibilities of caregiving. According to Family Caregiver Alliance, 40 to 70 percent of caregivers suffer from depression. Home Care Assistance found that 61 percent of family caregivers report significant emotional stress and 43 percent report physical stress from caring for a loved one with Alzheimer's.

> ❝ *You are just as important as your loved one.*

It's important to recognize that you are just as important as your loved one and that your thoughts and feelings matter. On any given day, your emotions can fluctuate; they can vacillate among acceptance, guilt, sadness, frustration, anger, loss, grief, disappointment, anxiety, relief, helplessness, isolation, depression, and resentment.

You're not alone. Virtually everyone experiences a range of emotions while caring for a loved one who changes and declines before their eyes. However, you can use your emotions to your benefit. Being in touch with your feelings is an opportunity for introspection and reassessing your circumstances. It allows you to gain new insights and different perspectives.

That said, it's not always easy to figure out what you're feeling. For example, depression can actually be anger — or anger can mask grief. You can use the emotions chart on the next page to help identify what you're feeling.

When you're experiencing strong emotions, ask yourself these three questions:

1. What are your emotions trying to tell you?
2. Why are you feeling this way?
3. What do you need to do differently?

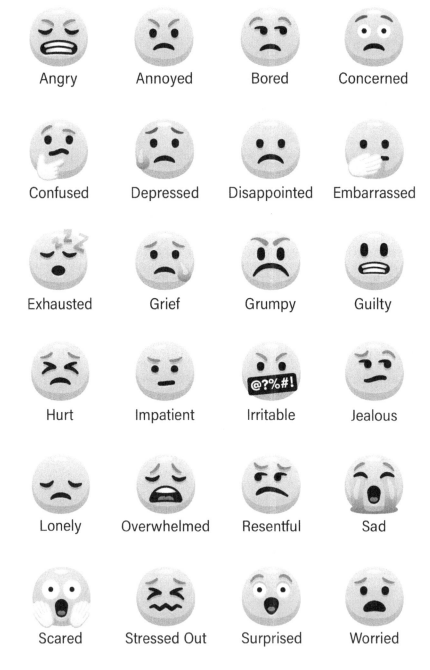

For example, DeShawn looks at the emotions chart and acknowledges that he's feeling overwhelmed and exhausted. He answers the three questions this way:

1. *What are your emotions trying to tell you?* I need to take a break. I need to get more sleep. I need more support.
2. *Why are you feeling this way?* I can't meet Debra's needs all the time. I'm expecting too much from myself.
3. *What do you need to do differently?* I need to ask family members and friends for help. I need respite care.

If you look at the chart and determine that you're feeling hurt and disappointed, you might answer the three questions this way:

1. *What are your emotions trying to tell you?* I'm taking what my loved one says and does personally.
2. *Why are you feeling this way?* My loved one blames me for everything.
3. *What do you need to do differently?* I need to detach from what my loved one says and remind myself that dementia is causing my loved one to behave this way.

If you look at the chart and determine that you're feeling stressed out and irritable, you might answer the three questions this way:

1. *What are your emotions trying to tell you?* I'm in over my head and worn out.
2. *Why are you feeling this way?* I don't have any help, and I don't get time for myself.

3. *What do you need to do differently?* I need to accept my limitations and ask for help. I need to take ten-minute timeouts and do something to comfort and nurture myself once a day.

If you look at the chart and determine that you're feeling angry and frustrated, you might answer the three questions this way:

1. *What are your emotions trying to tell you?* My patience is worn thin.

2. *Why are you feeling this way?* I can't manage my loved one's behaviors.

3. *What do you need to do differently?* Let go of what I can't control. Hire caregivers to help care for my loved one.

The answers to these three questions provide you with options that help you get through this journey and allow you to reflect on the time and quality of care you're providing to your loved one.

> *God, grant me the serenity to accept the things I cannot change, the courage to change the things I can, and the wisdom to know the difference.*
>
> — Serenity Prayer

The Serenity Prayer can be a helpful reminder to stay focused on the things you have control over and to let go of what you cannot control. The unfortunate reality is that you don't have control over dementia and its progression. However, you do have control over how you react to situations that occur as a result of dementia.

For example, when Debra gets angry at DeShawn for not telling her about the family picnic, DeShawn tries to convince Debra that he told her and that she doesn't remember. They go in circles, and DeShawn becomes increasingly exasperated. He realizes that he can't change what dementia is doing to Debra's brain, but he can change how he reacts. Since Debra is often forgetful about upcoming events, DeShawn comes up with a solution. He writes events on a whiteboard, leaves a sticky note by Debra's chair, and puts a note on the refrigerator as reminders. In addition, he writes down appointments and events on a calendar and then crosses them out once they've occurred.

Since Debra's memory is the problem, having a visual reminder can reduce how often she accuses DeShawn of not telling her about activities. And, instead of DeShawn trying to convince Debra of her memory loss and forgetfulness — something he has no control over — he instead puts his energy into finding solutions to the problem.

Dementia is a challenging disease to manage, observe, and navigate. It robs you and your loved one of time, experiences, and memories. Ignoring, suppressing, dismissing, or downplaying your feelings can make your journey harder. Knowing that you're not alone — that many others have walked this path and experienced what you're feeling — can be affirming and help normalize your journey.

Feeling Unappreciated and Resentful

It's common for caregivers to feel unappreciated by their loved one and other family members. Often, frustration builds and causes resentment. As the resentment builds, it takes a toll on you emotionally, physically, and mentally. Resentment is one of the primary causes of caregiver stress, burnout, and depression.

Unfortunately, you can't change your loved one. And it's unlikely that your family members are going to change. The only real option is to change your expectations of your loved one and your family members.

DeShawn does everything in his power to make sure Debra's needs are always met. He cooks, helps her with personal hygiene, takes her to all of her doctor's appointments, and is her constant companion. When Debra refuses to cooperate during bath time, DeShawn gets angry. He resents that his wife is being so difficult and is unappreciative of his efforts. He has put his life on hold to take care of her, and she never expresses appreciation for all that he does. As time goes on, DeShawn learns that he has to change his expectations of his wife and his family.

Changing your expectations of your loved one with dementia can be difficult. Start by acknowledging that dementia is a self-centered, self-absorbing, and all-consuming disease. Your loved one most likely is struggling to get through the day and probably isn't aware or capable of appreciating all that you do. Or, they might be appreciative but aren't able to express it properly. It's also possible that, in the early stages, your loved one struggles with acknowledging your help because their dependence on you reinforces their awareness of all the things that they can no longer do.

For example, Debra feels she can still drive, but DeShawn knows that this isn't the case. Every time he tells her that she needs to stop driving, the couple has a heated argument. In Debra's mind, she thinks she's a good driver and that DeShawn is trying to control her and take her independence away. The more DeShawn tries to convince Debra to stop driving, the more resentful she becomes. The more Debra refuses to listen and cooperate, the more resentful DeShawn becomes. In the end, they both resent each other.

Eventually, DeShawn realizes that he needs to change his expectations and find a solution. Instead of expecting Debra to acknowledge and appreciate his concern for her safety and that of others, DeShawn contacts her doctor and the DMV about his concerns. In addition, he disables Debra's car and makes arrangements to have her car towed and "taken to the shop for repairs." While Debra's car is in the shop, DeShawn does the driving and arranges for Debra's friends to pick her up and take her out.

By changing his expectations and placing the responsibility on the doctor and the DMV, DeShawn isn't the bad guy. He's able to deal with the driving issue without confronting Debra directly. Having the car towed allows DeShawn and Debra to work together and figure out ways to get around with only one car.

Your loved one might not be the only person who overlooks your efforts. There are several reasons why family members may take you for granted and not show appreciation. If you're the adult child, you may have always been the responsible one; family members may assume that caregiving is your role in the family. Family roles are established very early — often when we're children — and family dynamics can feel like they're set in stone. If you're a parent taking care of your spouse, your adult children may have difficulty admitting that their parent is declining. They may not express their appreciation because then they would have to come to terms with this reality.

For example, when DeShawn needs a break, he asks his stepchildren if they can come to the house and visit with their mother. They each have an excuse as to why they aren't available. DeShawn resents that his stepchildren only call when they need something and expect him to take care of Debra 24/7 with no help. Angry and frustrated, he confronts them. To his surprise, they say they don't feel comfortable visiting because they don't know what to talk about and how to have a conversation with their mother. Because Debra says things that aren't true or don't make sense, her children are uncomfortable visiting. It's easier for them to stay away.

Once DeShawn knows that his stepchildren aren't willing to visit, he changes his expectations. He realizes that he has to find other ways to get a break, so he begins scheduling friends to stop by and visit or take Debra out. He also hires a caregiver to come for four hours three times a week to provide companion care.

Another reason family members may not express their appreciation is that doing so reflects poorly on their inability to step up and help out. To acknowledge all that you're doing means admitting to themselves what they aren't doing.

Regardless of the reason, feeling unappreciated by your loved one with dementia or other family members can be disappointing, frustrating, infuriating, and upsetting. But the reality is that your loved one has a brain disease that causes them to disconnect from reality. And, the roles in your family are deeply ingrained and may not change.

When DeShawn feels resentful, it's a warning sign that he needs to step back and examine the underlying cause. For DeShawn, resentment is a red flag that his expectations are unrealistic or that he has a need that isn't being met. It may be that he's not taking enough time for himself or that he's putting others' needs ahead of his own. It's DeShawn's responsibility to deal with his resentment because that is the only thing he can control.

One way to do this is to stop expecting Debra to acknowledge and praise him for making three meals a day, doing the laundry, paying the bills, taking Debra to her appointments, and cleaning up after her. Instead, at the end of each day, DeShawn writes down in a notebook what he wishes Debra would say to him. He writes down, "Thank you for taking good care of me," "Thank you for all that you do for me," "Thank you for being there for me," and "Thank you for all of your love and support." At the end of each day, he says one of these phrases to himself.

DeShawn also has to adjust his expectations of his friends. He notices that they don't call as often, stop by to visit, or ask if he needs help. Rather than wait for them to contact him, DeShawn changes his expectations and accepts their limitations. Instead, he embraces the people who do call and joins a dementia caregiver support group. Joining the support group allows DeShawn to connect with other caregivers, get together with four of them regularly, and receive the support and validation he needs.

Taking care of a loved one with dementia can be all-consuming. When you feel unappreciated or under-appreciated, there are several ways to acknowledge and praise yourself for the hard work, love, compassion, care, and support you provide:

Keep a personal gratitude journal. Jot down messages of thanks for the things — big and small — that you do for your loved one.

Create a wish list. Write down how you'd like others to acknowledge your dedication, care, and love. Then do those things for yourself. For example, send yourself flowers as a form of acknowledgment, write yourself a thank you letter, or compose a poem of gratitude. Say to yourself what you wish other people would say to you, such as, "I'm an amazing person," or "I'm grateful to you for providing excellent care."

Make a recording. Record audio or video expressing gratitude for the things you do for your loved one, and then replay those messages when you need a lift.

Post on social media. Set up a curated friend list on Facebook of those you know who are supportive and post updates about the care and love you provide for your loved one.

Create affirmations. Using sticky notes, write down positive messages about your compassion, lovingness, and capacity to care. Then, put them in places you're likely to see them — your car visor, refrigerator, bathroom mirror, and so forth — to remind yourself of your value.

Connect with friends. Call or get together with a friend and share what you've done for your loved one and how proud you are of yourself.

Give yourself a gift. Buy yourself something special to acknowledge your hard work, such as a book or piece of jewelry that reminds you of the love, care, and compassion you're providing for your loved one.

Take a break. Ask a friend or family member to spend time with your loved one while you go out and celebrate yourself.

Join a support group. You can establish meaningful relationships while sharing and receiving validation and acceptance from people who understand what you are going through.

Feeling unappreciated and resentful is often part of the caregiver's journey. Counteracting that resentment is an essential component to preventing burnout and depression.

Dealing with Loss, Sadness, and Grief

As dementia changes your loved one's personality and robs them of their cognitive and physical abilities, it's natural for you to experience grief. While loss and sadness are typically associated with the grief experienced after someone passes away, the "dementia grief" experienced by caregivers begins long before your loved one dies. You may start grieving the day your loved one receives their diagnosis. It may begin when you start noticing unusual behaviors, such as forgetfulness, not paying their bills, mail stacking up, getting lost, increased confusion, poor judgment, or putting items in awkward places. These feelings continue as you watch them slowly decline.

Questions that often emerge when experiencing loss, sadness, and grief are:

- What do I do with my feelings of sadness and loss?
- How do I deal with my grief at the same time I'm taking care of my loved one?
- Does the sadness ever go away?
- Watching my loved one decline makes me very sad, and the loss is so profound – what do I do with these feelings?
- How do I deal with my feelings of anger and sadness at the same time?

It's common to have these thoughts and feelings. For example, DeShawn has slowly been adapting to Debra's gradual decline. One day, he receives notification that he's won an award. He can't wait to tell Debra. As he shares his excitement, DeShawn notices that Debra has a blank stare and puzzled look on her face. At that moment, it hits him that the person he has shared everything with isn't there. DeShawn breaks down and cries because he misses his best friend and the intimacy and companionship they shared. It brings to the surface the underlying loneliness and sadness he feels.

Just as the progression of dementia is unique to each person, so too is the caregiver's grieving process. Typically, dementia grief involves five stages: denial, anger, guilt, sadness, and acceptance. However, the process isn't linear. Caregivers go back and forth among the different stages at various times throughout the dementia journey. Most likely, you'll find yourself fluctuating from one stage to another depending on how your loved one is doing.

> *Grief is the process of accepting the unacceptable.*

Characteristics of the five stages of dementia grief include:

Denial

- Feeling numb, experiencing disbelief, and hoping the diagnosis is a mistake;
- Wishing for a treatment plan (for example, diet, exercise, medication, or herbs) to cure your loved one;
- Expecting your loved one to do better than others who have dementia;
- Convincing yourself that your loved one hasn't changed, and instead telling yourself they're just having a bad day; and
- Minimizing, ignoring, or dismissing problematic behaviors and symptoms.

Anger

- Being impatient and frustrated with your loved one or yourself;
- Losing your temper and raising your voice;
- Feeling annoyed that you have to deal with your loved one's behavioral, physical, and cognitive changes;
- Resenting family members who are unwilling or unable to help with caregiving responsibilities;
- Becoming extremely upset that dementia has turned your life upside down;
- Feeling isolated and trapped by the relentless demands of being a caregiver; and
- Having little or no tolerance for others' opinions and advice.

Guilt

- Feeling badly about not being able to fulfill the expectations and demands you've placed on yourself;
- Constructing judgmental "should" statements, such as, "I should be more compassionate and understanding," "I shouldn't get frustrated and angry," "I should be able to handle this on my own," or "I should visit them every day, but I don't want to;"
- Condemning yourself for wanting to do things or doing things that your loved one can no longer do;

- Feeling that you're letting your loved one down if you're unable to continue caring for them on your own;
- Beating yourself up for wanting this journey to end and the suffering to be over;
- Regretting aspects of your pre-dementia relationship, such as wishing you'd spent more time with your loved one; and
- Wishing you would have been more attentive or kind to your loved one prior to their diagnosis.

Sadness

- Experiencing sorrow that your loved one is drifting away from you;
- Crying frequently;
- Withdrawing from family, friends, and social activities;
- Feeling isolated and alone;
- Feeling depressed;
- Holding back tears so your loved one, family, and friends don't see you cry; and
- Feeling that you're at the end of your rope and can't go on like this.

Acceptance

- Living in the present moment and coming to terms with the reality that your loved one has dementia;
- Finding deeper meaning in the dementia journey;
- Awareness and acceptance of your feelings and emotions;
- Giving yourself permission to have a sense of humor and expressing it without feeling guilty;
- Acknowledging your limitations and accepting that you can't do this alone; and
- Asking for and accepting help from others.

The dementia grieving process also involves coming to terms with loss. For example, DeShawn is experiencing the loss of his wife, best friend, and partner. He's losing companionship, intimacy, and the future he envisioned for him and Debra.

Depending on your circumstances, you may feel a variety of losses:

- Loss of the relationship you once had with your loved one;
- Loss of companionship, support, or intimacy with your loved one;
- Loss of someone with whom to talk things over;
- Loss of fun and laughter with your loved one;
- Loss of acknowledging and celebrating special occasions with your loved one by your side;
- Loss of doing activities together;

- Loss of your previous lifestyle;
- Loss of your freedom;
- Loss of control over your life;
- Loss of the future you imagined; and
- Loss of financial security.

You might feel as though you don't have time to deal with your losses. After all, you have to do so much to take care of your loved one. Still, all of these losses add up to grief, which can show up in unexpected ways. If you're feeling depressed, angry, or guilty, the underlying issue may be loss. The same holds true if you're having trouble sleeping or experiencing other physical symptoms. It is crucial to identify your losses, acknowledge your feelings, and let yourself grieve and process the changes in your life.

Ambiguous Loss and Anticipatory Grief

> *Alzheimer's disease is often referred to as "The Long Goodbye."*

The kind of loss, sadness, and grief that dementia caregivers experience is often referred to as "ambiguous loss" and "anticipatory grief." These are two sides of the same coin. Unlike the single loss experienced when a loved one passes away, you experience multiple losses as your loved one changes and declines. While they are physically present, their mental or emotional state may be different than normal.

As Debra's cognitive functioning declines, DeShawn feels that he's losing pieces of her while she's alive. That's why Alzheimer's disease is often referred to as "The Long Goodbye." This ambiguous loss repeatedly occurs throughout the dementia journey as your loved one declines. DeShawn feels a strong sense of loss when he is sitting next to Debra and she can't carry on a rational conversation or doesn't make eye contact when he's talking to her or she's talking to him.

DeShawn's ambiguous loss also surfaces when Debra has moments of clarity and makes sense for a short period of time. It is hard for DeShawn not to think that, if she can do this every once in a while, she should be able to do it all of the time. Then, when Debra returns to her confused state, it triggers DeShawn's feelings of loss, sadness, and disappointment. This is called renewed grief.

Ambiguous loss can be difficult to recognize as grief because so much of your time and energy are spent dealing with caregiving's overwhelming demands and responsibilities. Your feelings get pushed aside. Yet, part of surviving this journey is allowing yourself to grieve the losses along the way and finding new and meaningful ways to make up for those losses.

There are varying degrees of anticipatory grief. You grieve because you miss who your loved one was prior to dementia. The sense of loss is profound, the change in roles is complex, and you may question your value and purpose in life. Caregivers are often in the position of making difficult decisions while living in fear of what lies ahead. For example, DeShawn worries about how long Debra will live and how the disease will affect them financially. This anticipatory grief also surfaces when DeShawn wonders if he can care for his wife at home and how long he'll be able to do so. His anxiety about

Debra's care is ongoing. It intensifies when DeShawn concludes that he can no longer take care of her at home by himself and needs to place her in a care community or hire in-home care assistance.

When you're caring for a loved one with dementia, sadness and loneliness come with the territory. It's important to acknowledge that loss and grief are normal and can be healing. These strategies may help you throughout your journey:

Identify and process your feelings. Instead of trying to push down the uncomfortable feelings, allow yourself to acknowledge them. Write in a journal, craft poems, recite prayers, create rituals, or draw or paint images.

Focus on what your loved one can do. Try to find peace and joy in the little things they can still do, whether it's sweeping, cleaning, stacking, counting, holding hands, or hugging you. Celebrate those moments.

Ask for assistance and emotional support. Talking about your feelings can be incredibly cathartic. Share your feelings and thoughts with a trusted family member, a close friend, a support group, a spiritual or religious leader, a dementia consultant, or a licensed professional therapist.

Stay in touch with the outside world. A common dementia caregiver pitfall is isolating yourself from family and friends. As your time and energy become increasingly dominated by caregiving duties, enjoyable activities drift away. Treating yourself to an afternoon or evening out with friends can relieve some of the sadness and loss.

Be good to yourself. Taking care of yourself in difficult times is hard. Accept that you may feel good one day and bad the next. Carve out time to do whatever is nurturing and comforting for you, like listening to music, watching favorite movies, going for walks, or playing solitaire.

Take one day at a time. No two days are alike. Caring for someone with dementia varies from day to day, and so does the grieving process. Living in the present with self-awareness allows you to acknowledge and process your loss, sadness, and grief.

Try to find meaning in the dementia journey. Take time to reflect on what you're learning about yourself and your relationship with your loved one. You're confronted with and learning to navigate many changes. Think about how those changes are having a positive and meaningful impact on you as a person, your relationships, and your life. Maybe you're learning to let go of the little things, take one day at a time, choose your battles, live in the moment, be patient, accept what you can't control, or laugh more. Perhaps you're learning the true meaning of unconditional love.

Create new rituals. Meet your loved one on their level and find new and meaningful ways to connect with them. Maybe it's smiling at one another, holding hands, laughing about silly things, listening to music together, singing songs, sitting side by side in silence, eating chocolate cake, or reading a poem or prayer. Be gentle with yourself and treasure the love, care, and support you're providing during moments of togetherness.

Don't compare your sadness, loss, and grief. Your feelings and experience are your own. While others may walk a similar journey, your experience is unique. Several factors influence your feelings. These include the history of your relationship with your loved one, previous losses you've experienced, and how dementia is altering your loved one's personality, behaviors, and ability to function.

The Role of a Support Network

It is very difficult to travel the dementia caregiving journey alone. Creating a support network is a necessity. It's equally as important as getting your medical and legal documents in order. It's imperative to have family, friends, community services, spiritual advisors, and professional counselors to help you.

You may also want to consider attending a caregiver support group. Support groups normalize what you're going through while validating your feelings and emotions. Other caregivers provide suggestions for challenging and difficult situations. Meetings are informal, and you can choose to share or not share depending on your comfort level. The camaraderie is invaluable, and you quickly learn that you're not alone.

Questions that often emerge about a support network are:

- Why is establishing a support network so important?
- How do I establish a support network?
- Can friends and family be a part of the support network?
- Where do I start?

There are many reasons to be hesitant about reaching out to family, friends, and others to help you. Creating a support network can be uncomfortable. Initially, DeShawn found it difficult because it was an admission that he needed help. In addition, he didn't want to impose on others, was afraid that people would think he was weak, and didn't want to deal with the potential disappointment of people letting him down.

In DeShawn's mind, these were all good reasons not to ask for help. But, in reality, it got to the point that he couldn't care for Debra alone. He had to ask for help. In hindsight, he realizes that it would have been so much easier had he sought support in advance rather than waiting until he reached his breaking point. If he had acknowledged and accepted his limitations sooner, he would have been ahead of the game. If he knew about the available resources, he wouldn't have felt as distressed and desperate when he needed help.

The bottom line is that it's never too early to create a support network, and it's never too late to develop a support network. Your support network will change as your needs change and as your loved one's needs change. Ultimately, your support network will become part of your care plan and part of your survival guide.

> **Creating a Support Network in Three Steps**
> 1. Write down the types of help you want or need.
> 2. Make a list of available resources.
> 3. Utilize those resources and ask for help.

To jump-start this process, make two columns on a sheet of paper or a spreadsheet. At the top of the sheet, write, "My Dementia Support Network."

Step 1: Title the left column "Help I Need." Next, list the tasks you don't want to do, don't like to do, or aren't able to do. For example, you might list:

- Housework;
- Cooking meals;
- Dressing my loved one;
- Driving my loved one;
- Keeping my loved one occupied during the day;
- Assisting my loved one in the bathroom and cleaning up after them;
- Organizing papers and files;
- Bathing my loved one; or
- Running errands.

Recognizing and accepting your limitations is liberating and healthy. You simply cannot do everything alone, and the sooner you acknowledge this, the easier this journey will be on you and your loved one.

Putting your needs on the back burner significantly increases your chances of caregiver isolation, burnout, stress, and depression. According to researchers, up to 60 percent of Alzheimer's caregivers exhibit symptoms of clinical depression.

Caregiver Stress, Burnout, and Depression Scale

Over the past two weeks, how often have you experienced the following?

- Stress
- Burnout
- Depression

Take the survey on the following pages to gauge your level of stress, burnout, or depression.

Download Free Resources

Scan this QR code or visit tamianastasia.com/caregivers to download the logs referenced in this book.

Caregiver Stress, Burnout, and Depression Scale

	Not at all	Several days	More than half the days	Nearly every day
Caregiver Stress				
Trouble falling or staying asleep, or sleeping too much	0	1	2	3
Poor appetite or overeating	0	1	2	3
Wanting to hurt yourself or person you're caring for	0	1	2	3
Feeling irritable, frustrated, or angry	0	1	2	3
Feeling anxious, restless, or out of control	0	1	2	3
Caregiver Burnout				
Unrelenting emotional and physical exhaustion	0	1	2	3
Difficulty remembering, concentrating, or making decisions	0	1	2	3

Feeling sick	0	1	2	3
Feeling worthless, overwhelmed, guilty, or inadequate	0	1	2	3
Little interest in previous activities once enjoyed	0	1	2	3
Caregiver Depression				
Withdrawing from family and friends	0	1	2	3
Feeling sad, hopeless, or helpless	0	1	2	3
Not seeking support or asking for help	0	1	2	3
Thoughts that you would be better off dead	0	1	2	3
Crying easily or for no reason at all	0	1	2	3
Totals				
	A	B	C	D	A+B+C+D

If stress and burnout aren't dealt with, they can turn into depression. You can use this table to gauge your level of stress, burnout, or depression:

None	0-7
Mild	8-14
Moderate	15-21
Moderately severe	22-28
Severe	29-45

If your score is 15 or more, you should consider seeking professional help and increasing your support network.

Step 2: Title the right column "My Support Network." Next to each task or item listed in the left column, write down the names of family members and friends, along with professional, community, or faith-based services that might be able to fill that need — either currently or further down the road. Also, list their contact information.

For example, DeShawn's list includes:

HELP I NEED	MY SUPPORT NETWORK
Meals	Marge, 123-4567
	Good Faith Church, 234-5678
	Pedro, private chef, 345-6789
	Meals on Wheels, mealsonwheelsamerica.org
Groceries	Instacart, instacart.com
	Safeway pickup, Safeway.com
Housekeeping	Merry Maids, merrymaids.com
	Ask Jenny for referral, 111-2222
Respite Care	Sherry, 222-3333
	Jamie, 333-4444
	Grate Respite Care, 444-5555
Companionship (Debra)	Companion Care, 555-6666
	Sam & Joan, 222-7777
Emotional Support (DeShawn)	Tami Anastasia, tami@tamianastasia.com tamianastasia.com
	Rita Glendora, 777-8888
	Rev. Tom Doe, 888-9999
Bathing Assistance	Helpful In-Home Care, 999-1111
	Ask Betsy, 111-3333

While developing your support network, you may find that there's overlap in certain areas. For example, three friends may offer to help with meals. Having multiple people willing to help out with the same task allows you to rotate among them. This prevents helper burnout and provides you with backup in case someone has to cancel. The bottom line is that you can never have too much support — the more extensive your support network, the better.

Resources to consider including in your support network are:

- Caregiver support group;
- Counselor or therapist;
- Doctor or geriatrician;
- Geriatric care manager;
- Spiritual leader, guide, or mentor;
- Community services resources;
- Home care agency for companion and personal care;
- Activity specialist;
- Home safety service for home modifications;
- Adult day program or senior center;
- Childcare provider;
- Carpooling;
- Transportation service;
- Meal delivery service;
- Elder law attorney;

- Family elder mediator;
- Human resources department for Family Medical Leave Act, leave of absence, or employee assistance program;
- Assisted living and memory care community;
- Respite grants;
- Long-term care insurance;
- Veterans Administration;
- In-home support service;
- Area agency on aging; and
- Medicare.

Step 3: The next step is to reach out and actually ask for help. Utilize your resources as soon as possible. Try not to wait until your responsibilities become overwhelming or a crisis occurs. Having a support network in place better prepares you to deal with your loved one's needs and challenges — both now and in the future. Most importantly, it gives you a break from day-to-day demands and responsibilities and provides you with the support you need and deserve.

> *Your goal as a caregiver is to survive this journey the best you can, and not at the expense of your physical, mental, and emotional well-being.*

Remember that family members, neighbors, friends, and community organizations are willing to help you, but they don't know what you need unless you tell them. For example, DeShawn makes the mistake of asking friends to drop off meals, and he ends up with four tuna casseroles sitting in the refrigerator. The problem? DeShawn and Debra don't like tuna. The key is to be specific and ask for what you want and need. For meal preparation, provide a list of dietary preferences and restrictions. For a trip to the store, send a list with brand names and quantities. Your helper will be happy to pick up what you want, and you'll be glad to get what you need.

When you ask people from your support network for help, capitalize on each person's strengths. For example, ask people who love to cook to bring you meals. Ask those who enjoy running errands to go to the grocery store, post office, and pharmacy. Contact those who like to socialize and ask them to spend a few hours with your loved one. People want to pitch in, and they'll be much more enthusiastic about helping you if you ask them to do things they enjoy. You may also want to consider assigning people specific tasks and setting up a schedule.

If setting schedules and assigning tasks to your support network feels overwhelming, consider utilizing an online tool designed to coordinate support. Type the term "care calendar" into Google to see what's available and find an option that works for you. These online tools allow you to invite people to be part of your support network and post tasks that need to be performed. Those in your network then volunteer for specific tasks. With a care calendar, everyone is on the same page, and you don't have to worry about following up with each individual.

Taking care of someone living with dementia can be a long, demanding, and challenging journey. To make your time with them as loving, compassionate, joyful, and meaningful as possible, you need all of the help and support you can get. Ultimately, you're creating a care plan and a survival guide, both of which are essential for your emotional, physical, and mental well-being.

Caregiver Guilt

Giving yourself permission to take care of yourself goes hand in hand with creating a support network. All too often, however, caregiver guilt interferes with self-care.

You may feel guilty when you:

- Want to take time out for yourself;
- Want a break from being a caregiver;
- Can't meet all of your loved one's needs;
- Feel you're letting your loved one down;
- Make difficult decisions for your loved one;
- Lose your temper;
- Can't honor your promises or marriage vows;
- Are tired and don't want to be a caregiver anymore;
- Upset your loved one; or
- Feel like you're not doing a good job taking care of your loved one.

These are normal feelings when caring for a loved one with dementia. Most of us are raised to feel that we are responsible for taking care of others before taking care of ourselves. There's an underlying assumption that we're selfish if we take care of ourselves first.

Throughout our lives, we are repeatedly subjected to messages that reinforce this view, such as:

- Other people's needs more important than our own needs.
- We are responsible for taking care of others at all times.
- We should know how to meet our loved one's needs.
- If we fall short of meeting their needs, we aren't fulfilling our responsibilities.
- Asking for help is an admission of failure.
- Feeling overwhelmed, frustrated, or angry is a sign of weakness.

> *Guilt implies that you are doing something wrong. It places all of the blame on you, and it puts all of the responsibility on you. Dementia is responsible for what you and your loved one are going through. Guilt is a useless and unproductive emotion in dementia care.*

Caregivers may feel guilty about things they've said and done, wanting to run away, wanting it to be over, bringing in outside support, or placing their loved one in a care community. For example, DeShawn questions whether he is doing a good job caring for Debra because she gets upset when he leaves the house without her and when caregivers come to care for her. DeShawn struggles, knowing that he's doing what he has to do and that it goes against her wishes. He brings this up in his support group, and the unanimous feedback is, "You're doing a great job caring for your wife. You're attentive to her needs, and you try to make her happy. Debra getting upset doesn't mean you're doing something wrong. She has dementia and doesn't understand that you're doing what's best for her and you." When DeShawn starts questioning himself, he reminds himself of what those in his support group said.

Familial and cultural messages cause caregivers to fall into three common guilt traps:

- Wanting approval and support from their loved one;
- Having unrealistic expectations of their capacity for caregiving; and
- Comparing themselves to others.

Understandably, caregivers want validation that they're doing the right thing, but their loved ones can't provide that approval. It's easy to fall into the guilt trap of wanting approval from your loved one for the decisions you make. But your loved one's brain cannot understand or accept some of those decisions, leaving you distressed.

Given the circumstances, you have to know in your heart that you're doing what is right. If your loved one disagrees, disapproves, or gets angry, it doesn't mean that you're doing something wrong. It means that you're making decisions for them that they can't make for themselves. This is a very difficult position to be in. Sometimes, what is in their best interest is doing what is best for you. Sometimes, what is in their best interest is doing what goes against their wishes.

You start this journey wanting to respect and honor your loved one's wishes and the promises you made, but dementia may not allow it. You're not at fault. Dementia ultimately dictates the choices and decisions you have to make. You're doing what you must in order to provide the necessary care that dementia requires. Remember that you have to be the voice of reason and that every decision you make is in the best interest of your loved one.

The second guilt trap that caregivers fall into is having unrealistic expectations of themselves. As a caregiver, the degree to which you feel guilty is often based on how you or others measure your performance. In other words, the guilt you feel is built on your perceptions or the perceptions of others — whether you or others think you're living up to the expectations and demands of caring for your loved one.

The problem is that this thinking ignores or dismisses your needs and doesn't consider the extraordinary amount of care that a person living with dementia requires as the disease progresses. When you experience caregiver burnout and can no longer meet the responsibilities of caring for your loved one, you feel guilty. And the more you feel guilty, the more pressure you put on yourself to step it up. At this point, being a caregiver comes at the expense of your physical, mental, and emotional well-being. Caregiving becomes a vicious cycle of stress, burnout, and depression.

> *Dementia requires that you take care of both yourself and your loved one.*

To avoid this trap, pay attention to your limitations, as well as the warning signs of caregiver stress, burnout, and depression. Give yourself permission to ask for help and take frequent breaks from being a caregiver. Stay connected to family and friends and get support when you need it. Lower your expectations so that they are realistic and meet your needs.

You know your expectations are unrealistic when you use the word "should." Pay attention to how many times a day you say to yourself, "I should," and then feel bad because you don't do or say something. "Shoulds" are unrealistic expectations you place on yourself and lead to guilt. Your expectations may be self-imposed or develop from messages ingrained by your family or culture.

When caring for a loved one living with dementia, there are many conflicting emotions — grief, loss, frustration, anger, resentment, sadness, and disappointment. Your capacity for caring for your loved one depends on how you're feeling. Shift the focus from what you think you "should" be doing and develop a "can do" attitude. A "can do" attitude converts unrealistic expectations into realistic expectations. It empowers you, gives you a sense of control, and helps with prioritizing and time management.

To help you make this shift, replace your "should" statements with what you can, will, or want to do. Here are examples:

Should Statement Unrealistic Expectations	Can Do Attitude Realistic Expectations
I "should" be able to do this on my own.	I "can" visit my parents in the afternoon. I "will" ask family and friends for help. I "want" to have dinner with my family.
I "should" be more patient.	I "can" be patient when I'm not in a rush. I "will" count to three before I say anything. I "want" to work on taking time out for myself.

Converting your "should" statements turns them into action items — things that you can, will, and want to do. You become proactive rather than passive.

The third guilt trap is comparing yourself to others. No two people with dementia are the same, and no two caregivers are the same. Moreover, each relationship is unique and has its own dynamics. To avoid this trap, examine why you're comparing yourself to others and what it is that you need. For example, do you need:

- Reassurance that you're doing the right thing?
- Acknowledgment that you're doing a good job?
- Permission to try something new or different?
- Validation for the way you feel?
- To know if your situation is better or worse than others?
- Praise, appreciation, or approval for all that you're doing?

Once you can identify your needs, give back to yourself what you seek. For example, tell yourself you're doing a good job or that you're doing the right thing, and give yourself permission to try something different if what you're doing isn't working.

If you're comparing yourself to others, pay attention to why you do this and how it affects you. Comparing yourself to others can make you feel worse about yourself and your situation because you may be self-critical and self-judgmental. If you compare yourself to others to gauge how you're doing, consider it a red flag. Let it be a learning opportunity. Ask yourself, "What is this telling me or teaching me?"

Know that your situation is very common, and normalize it instead of being judgmental or critical. For example, when DeShawn talks to a friend who cared for his mother with dementia, he immediately starts to compare himself to his friend. DeShawn tells his friend how inadequate and unprepared he feels. His friend tells

DeShawn that this is normal. "You learn by doing. You learn by trial and error, and mistakes are opportunities to learn." He says that DeShawn needs to accept that he's doing the best he can. Later, when DeShawn starts comparing himself to others and starts feeling inadequate, he reminds himself that he's learning as he goes along.

When you're feeling guilty, ask yourself:

- Why am I feeling guilty?
- What do I need to change so I don't feel guilty?
- What do I need to do differently to lessen the guilt?
- What would make me feel better?

Guilt is not a productive emotion in dementia care. Feeling guilty isn't going to make the dementia go away. Feeling guilty isn't going to make you a better caregiver. Guilt is a vicious cycle that erodes your self-esteem and increases your stress level. Replace guilt with compassion. You're working very hard to provide the best care possible. You're doing the best you can. No one is perfect, and there is no ideal roadmap.

The good news is that guilt is a learned response and can be reduced. If you change your reactions to the circumstances that make you feel guilty, your guilt will decrease and your struggle will lessen.

Compassionate Self-Understanding

Compassionate self-understanding occurs when you replace guilt and negative self-talk with non-judgmental self-talk. It involves acknowledging your imperfections and limitations in ways that are loving and compassionate. At its essence, compassionate self-understanding is speaking to yourself the way you talk to a dear friend who is self-critical or self-judgmental.

For example, DeShawn blames himself when he checks on the laundry and Debra falls in the living room. He keeps apologizing to her and tells himself, "I should have known better than to leave her by herself." His wife didn't get hurt, but DeShawn feels responsible for not being in the same room with her. The reality is that Debra typically sits in her chair and doesn't try to get up. DeShawn couldn't have predicted that this was going to happen. Instead of blaming himself for what happened, DeShawn changes his self-talk to, "Accidents happen, and I didn't cause Debra to fall." But this incident brings to DeShawn's attention that he needs more assistance with taking care of his wife.

Guilt makes you feel trapped, stuck, and powerless, whereas compassionate self-understanding allows you to reflect, respond, and adapt to your circumstances. Compassionate self-understanding is empowering and can provide you with valuable insights.

> *Of all the judgments we pass in life, none is more important than the judgment we pass on ourselves.*
> — Nathaniel Branden

For example, DeShawn feels extremely guilty when he wants to take a break. He thinks he's being selfish. After examining his guilt, DeShawn realizes that it's difficult spending time with Debra because it's depressing and emotionally painful to watch her decline. It's not that he's selfish; it's that his heart is breaking. Once DeShawn realizes this, he practices self-compassion, forgives himself, and finds ways to cope with his sadness. For example, he makes arrangements for friends to interact with Debra so he doesn't feel like he's abandoning her. And, in return, this frees him up to do things with his wife that make him feel better about the time he does spend with her. As a result, DeShawn is more patient and relaxed when they play games together, when they eat meals together, and when it's time to get ready for bed. Giving himself permission to support his well-being shifts DeShawn's focus from the quantity of time he spends with Debra to the quality of time they spend together.

An excellent first step in moving away from guilt and toward compassionate self-understanding is to write down all of the things that make you feel guilty and then write down what you would say to a friend if they vocalized those same feelings. You would go to great lengths to be supportive, kind, compassionate, and understanding with your friend. Do the same with yourself.

Another important step is to acknowledge that your feelings are normal. It's common for those taking care of someone living with dementia to say:

- I have negative feelings and thoughts about my loved one.
- I feel angry, exhausted, overwhelmed, and resentful.
- I feel isolated, sad, lonely, and frustrated.
- I feel obligated to take care of my loved one.
- I feel I'm letting my loved one down.
- I don't think that I'm a good caregiver.
- I want this responsibility to be over.

- I hate being a caregiver.
- I want my loved one's suffering to end.
- I want to move on with my life.

Given that these are normal caregiver feelings, try to shift your focus away from feeling guilty and toward figuring out how to cope with these thoughts and feelings.

One way to replace guilt with compassionate self-understanding is by changing your beliefs about and expectations of yourself as a caregiver. You have limitations, and you don't always know your loved one's needs, especially if they aren't able to articulate them. And your needs are just as important as their needs. As a matter of fact, your needs are even more important because how you take care of yourself affects how you care for your loved one.

Examples of compassionate self-talk phrases are:

- I try to do what's right, but sometimes, I make mistakes.
- I'm not a failure. I'm learning as I go.
- Patience is a learned skill, and I'm working on it.
- I will have negative thoughts and feelings, but that doesn't make me a bad person.
- I'm doing the best I can. Some days are better than others.
- I make decisions with the best of intentions.

Start changing your beliefs and expectations of yourself as a caregiver by posting the PACE Caregiver Principles to your bathroom mirror, the refrigerator, a kitchen cabinet, or another place where you'll read it daily.

PACE Caregiver Principles

- My feelings and needs are just as important as my loved one's feelings and needs.
- It's okay for me to ask for help because I cannot do it alone.
- I have limitations, and I need to respect and honor those limitations.
- The decisions I make are made with the best of intentions.
- I am as significant as the person I'm taking care of.
- Taking care of myself is not an act of selfishness – it's an act of kindness.
- I need to accept and forgive myself for what I cannot or do not want to do.
- I'm doing the best that I can, given the circumstances.

The PACE Caregiver Principles remind you that taking care of yourself is essential and that you need to find a balance between taking care of your loved one and taking care of yourself.

> *Dementia may change your loved one, but don't let it destroy your self-confidence, self-esteem, value, and purpose.*

Caring for someone living with dementia is incredibly taxing. Many caregivers find it challenging to take time out for themselves because of the demands and responsibilities placed upon them. Some feel guilty or selfish when they take time for themselves. Others feel trapped and don't have time to take a break. Many feel they don't have reliable help or don't have the financial resources to hire help. Even though the thought of taking time out for yourself may feel impossible, it's the very thing you need to do.

While it can be overwhelming to think about taking care of yourself, it is essential to make a conscious effort to factor in time for yourself daily. Start by thinking in increments of ten minutes. Ask yourself, "What can I do for ten minutes that will make me feel good?" If it turns out that you can take more than ten minutes, that's a bonus.

Ten minutes is just enough time to give yourself a break from the intensity, demands, and responsibilities of caregiving. There are many activities that you can do for ten minutes that support your physical, mental, and emotional well-being.

> " Letting your health suffer isn't going to make your loved one better.

Use your first ten-minute block to write down a list of things you can do in ten minutes that are nurturing, comforting, or pleasurable. Here are ideas to get you started:

- Eating a snack;
- Sipping coffee or tea;
- Flipping through a magazine;
- Walking around the block;
- Sitting outdoors;

- Calling or texting a friend;
- Knitting;
- Journaling;
- Singing;
- Listening or dancing to music;
- Cutting flowers from the garden;
- Working on a puzzle;
- Meditation or yoga;
- Closing your eyes;
- Organizing a drawer;
- Cuddling with the dog; and
- Drawing or coloring.

Being a caregiver can be incredibly rewarding, but it shouldn't be at the expense of your well-being. Letting your health suffer isn't going to make your loved one better.

Action Plan: Understanding Your Feelings

1. Have the difficult conversation with your loved one and your family about dementia care options.

2. Give yourself permission to feel all of your feelings – joy and sadness, love and resentment, happiness and grief.

3. Make a list of people to include in your support network during your caregiving journey. Make it a priority to connect with at least one person each day, whether it's a quick check-in via text, a longer phone chat, or an in-person visit.

4. Mini-breaks will get you through the day. Create a list of enjoyable things you can do in ten-minute increments. Consider writing each on a slip of paper and putting the slips of paper in a container. When you need a break, pick one from the container for an element of surprise.

PACE
E = Empower Yourself

> P = Permission for Trial and Error
> A = Acknowledge Their Reality
> C = Compassionate Care
> **E = Empower Yourself**

Tracy raised Emma, her only child, as a single mom in Des Moines, Iowa. After Emma graduated from high school, she moved to Chicago to attend college and never looked back. Emma established a flourishing career as a museum curator and loved the vibrancy of the Windy City. A year after Tracy was diagnosed with dementia, Emma reluctantly left Chicago and moved home to care for her mother. While she knows it's her responsibility to care for her mother, Emma mourns both the loss of the mother she knew and the loss of her life in Chicago.

Educating Yourself

Dementia doesn't come with a set of instructions, so it's up to you to put on your detective's cap and unlock the mysteries of how the disease impacts both you and your loved one.

One of the greatest gifts we have is our observational ability, but we often don't use that ability to our advantage. As unpredictable as dementia is, there are times when your loved one's behavior occurs for a reason. If you can identify patterns, triggers, or causes, you can take preventative measures to decrease the frequency of the behavior or possibly extinguish the behavior altogether.

One of the best strategies you can use is documenting your loved one's moods and behaviors in an observational log. Here's a sample:

Observational Log

Date / Time	Event	Potential Trigger	Observation	Next Time, Try...
Monday March 15, 3:00 PM	Mom hit me.	Helping her pull down her pants in the bathroom.	She didn't like it when I tried helping her pull down her pants.	Demonstrating how to do it and have her pull down her own pants.
Wednesday March 17, 11:00 AM	Mom yelled at me.	Told her I couldn't take her to see her best friend because she's deceased.	She didn't believe her best friend was deceased.	Not telling her that her friend has died; tell her that her friend is away on vacation.

Download Free Resources

Scan this QR code or visit tamianastasia.com/caregivers to download the logs referenced in this book.

Occasionally, Tracy kicks her daughter out of the house, screams at her, and tells her not to return. Since this only happens sporadically, Emma starts to keep an observational log where she writes down the sequence of events. Emma writes down the exact words her mother verbalizes, Tracy's tone of voice, what Emma is doing when her mother has an outburst, and what Emma is wearing when her mother starts screaming at her. She also writes down the day of the week and the time of day. After keeping track of this for six weeks, a pattern emerges. It turns out that Tracy reacts this way every time Emma wears something red — a red hat, red shirt, or red jacket. Emma would never have figured this out if she hadn't written down her observations.

One of the best ways to educate yourself is to write down your observations about your loved one's behavior or mood. This is beneficial for you and your loved one's doctor. Documenting your observations allows you to process information about their behavior more objectively. Maintaining a cumulative record enables you to see patterns and changes over time. Finally, writing down your observations lets you identify potential triggers that may be preventable or treatable.

> The first step toward change is awareness.
> The second step is acceptance.
> — Nathaniel Branden

Here is a list of the most common preventable or treatable causes of behavior or mood changes, along with what action to take:

1. **Urinary tract infection.** UTIs can cause sudden behavior changes, restlessness, hallucinations, increased confusion, delusions, irritability, withdrawal, agitation, or weakness. If untreated, a UTI can become a severe threat to your loved one's health. Call the doctor. To diagnose a UTI, they'll ask for a urine sample. If the test confirms a UTI, the doctor will prescribe an antibiotic.

2. **Pain or physical discomfort.** Pay attention if your loved one repeatedly complains, moans, winces, paces, holds or rubs an area, or is agitated. If they have a history of pain, such as a bad back, arthritis, or the aftermath of a fall, follow up with their doctor and ask about pain management options.

3. **Sundown syndrome.** If your loved one gets fidgety, anxious, or agitated in the late afternoon or evening, or if they have mood changes or increased confusion, they may be experiencing sundown syndrome. If so, keep the house well-lit and engage your loved one in a stimulating or enjoyable activity during that time period.

4. **Medication side effects.** Medications are a common cause of sudden mood and behavioral changes. Write down changes in medication and note if there's a change in your loved one's baseline mood or behavior. If so, contact their doctor and explain the sequence of events and your observations.

5. **Dehydration.** Dehydration is common in people with dementia. It can cause increased confusion, behavioral changes, nausea, muscle cramping, and dizziness. If possible, get your loved one to drink two quarts of fluids per day. If they refuse

to drink water, consider giving them juice, milk, coffee, tea, soup, ice cream, popsicles, and fruit. Dehydration can lead to serious health issues, including constipation, falls, hallucinations, and urinary tract infections. It can even result in hospitalization.

6. **Thyroid imbalance.** When the thyroid is overactive (hyperthyroidism) or underactive (hypothyroidism), it can cause memory loss, difficulty concentrating, and similar dementia-like symptoms. A blood test can determine a thyroid imbalance.

7. **Hearing loss.** Hearing loss can contribute to increased confusion, frustration, and difficulty focusing. Have your loved one's hearing checked regularly, especially if they have hearing aids. If they refuse to wear their hearing aids, when you speak to them make sure to be at their eye level, face them directly, and speak slowly. A person may have hearing loss if they are more easily distracted or more confused than usual, turn up the volume on the television or radio, or can't follow what is said.

8. **Vision changes.** Suppose your loved one is falling or tripping more frequently, bumping into objects, reaching in the air because they're misjudging an object's distance, or lifting their feet exceptionally high for fear of stepping on an object. In that case, it could be due to changes in their vision. The field of vision can get as small as 12 inches for people with dementia. In addition, peripheral vision narrows and depth perception gets thrown off. As your loved one's vision changes, they may only see things directly in front of them. For example, they might eat what's in front of them but may leave

food on the outer part of their plate because they can't see it. Or, they may not be able to differentiate between a flat surface and a raised surface. To increase their safety, stand directly in front of them, use contrasting colors, pick up throw rugs, and increase the lighting in the house.

9. **Hunger.** Your loved one's mood or personality can change because they are hungry. Try to maintain a consistent meal schedule and provide snacks. Going for long periods without food can cause increased confusion, weakness, agitation, anxiety, irritability, and mood swings.

10. **Bathroom issues.** A person with dementia can become agitated, anxious, or frustrated when they soil their clothing and can't verbalize their discomfort. Check to see if they have had an accident and maintain a consistent bathroom schedule or routine.

11. **Your demeanor.** People with dementia are extremely sensitive to body language, facial expressions, and tone of voice. If your loved one's mood changes suddenly, they may be reacting to your behavior. Remember to slow down, speak softly, use a gentle touch, and smile encouragingly.

12. **Your words.** As the brain deteriorates, people with dementia experience severe memory loss and altered states of reality. They believe what their mind tells them rather than the objective truth. If you notice sudden anger, upset, or agitation, your loved one may be reacting to something you said. Avoid discussing topics that could be upsetting or that they don't understand.

> *The more knowledgeable you become, the more prepared you will be to deal with the challenges and demands that occur when taking care of a loved one with dementia.*

It's extremely important to document your loved one's behaviors. It's equally as important to educate yourself about your triggers. If you have past issues with your loved one, dementia will likely bring those issues to the surface. As a result, your buttons may be pushed. The more you become aware of your triggers, the better prepared you are to deal with the effects of dementia. Your loved one is not going to be able to change, but you can change how you react and cope with the circumstances of the disease.

To learn more about your triggers, write down your reactions to situations that are upsetting you, frustrating you, or making you angry. Emma's caregiver trigger log might look like the example on the next page.

Download Free Resources

Scan this QR code or visit tamianastasia.com/caregivers to download the logs referenced in this book.

Caregiver Observational Log

Date / Time	Event	Potential Trigger	Observation	Note to Self
Tuesday April 16, 3:00 PM	I got defensive.	Mom told me I looked like a tramp.	I felt like I wasn't good enough.	Don't react to comments about my clothing or appearance. Say, "Thank you for sharing your thoughts," and let it go.
Thursday April 18, 11:00 AM	I raised my voice.	Mom complained about my cooking.	I felt judged and criticized.	Don't take it personally. Give her something else to eat and put the leftovers away.
Saturday April 20, 1:00 PM	I threw a towel.	Mom was difficult when I tried to give her a bath.	I felt like she was manipulative and controlling so she could get her way.	Mom behaves this way because of dementia. Don't force a bath; try again a different day.

A variety of circumstances can trigger your reaction. When an event occurs, ask yourself if you are reacting to:

- What your loved one is saying: Are there specific words or topics that push your buttons?
- Their tone of voice: Is it harsh, timid, soft-spoken, insistent, insulting, or condescending?
- Paranoia: Is your loved one accusing you of hiding or stealing things?
- An uncooperative or difficult attitude: Are they refusing to change their clothes or shower, soiling themselves, or spilling food on themselves?
- The time of day: Is it morning, afternoon, evening, or bedtime?
- Being interrupted: Do they constantly interrupt you when you prepare a meal, work on a project, or clean the house?
- Feeling rushed: Are they slowing you down, taking too long, or getting distracted and not being compliant?
- Feeling embarrassed: Are they saying or doing inappropriate things in public?
- Their confusion: Are they mixing you up with someone else or unable to recognize you?
- An inability to communicate: Are they unable to comprehend what you're saying, being irrational, misinterpreting your words, or ignoring you?

- Clinginess: Are they joined to you at the hip, preventing you from having any space or personal time, or wanting to know where you are at all times?
- Repetitiveness: Are they asking the same question or saying the same thing over and over again?

These events are common for people living with dementia. When you can identify your triggers, you can prepare yourself to handle these situations and develop better coping skills. For example, Emma loses her temper when Tracy repeatedly asks, "Where are you going? When are you coming back?" This pushes Emma's buttons because, when she was younger, her mother was very controlling and critical. However, now the issue is that these are common questions asked by people with dementia. When Emma is aware that these questions are triggers, she can detach, refrain from reacting negatively, and formulate responses.

As Emma works through this process, she learns that Tracy asks these questions because she has an underlying fear of being left alone, abandoned, or forgotten. Understanding this through the lens of her mother's dementia, Emma responds by saying:

- "I'll be back soon. I'm going to the grocery store to pick up food for us to eat."
- "I'll be back in time for us to have dinner together."
- "I'm going for a walk. We'll eat lunch when I get back."
- "I'm going shopping. I'll bring back goodies for us to enjoy."

These responses comfort and reassure her mother. Tracy knows that Emma's coming back and that they will do something together when she returns. Even if her mother doesn't remember what Emma tells her, these responses are calming in the moment.

Emma also gets frustrated when Tracy falsely accuses Emma of hiding her mother's reading glasses. Emma either snaps at her mother or gets defensive. Once Emma realizes that this is another one of her triggers, she tries to understand the situation from a dementia perspective. Tracy feels out of control without her glasses and must have them nearby at all times. Once Emma is aware of this, she prepares three different responses she can use when this situation occurs:

- "I know it's important for you to have your glasses. I'll find them and bring them to you."
- "I'm sorry I misplaced your glasses. Where do you want me to put them when I find them?"
- "I know it's upsetting when you can't find your glasses. I know where they are."

Emma uses these phrases interchangeably and buys a few extra pairs of glasses so that, when Tracy accuses Emma, she can quickly grab a pair of backup glasses to give to her mother.

The most common items that go missing are reading glasses, remote controls, purses, and wallets. The best way to deal with missing items is to buy duplicates so that when your loved one hides the item, you immediately have a replacement to give them.

Remember that repetitive questions and accusations mask an underlying need. Rather than react, listen and try to figure out what the need might be. Once you can identify the need, you can develop interchangeable responses or actions to satisfy that need.

Educating yourself involves not only learning about dementia but also learning more about yourself. Understanding your triggers and your loved one's triggers allow you to develop appropriate responses that decrease caregiver stress.

Dealing with Other Family Members

Often, an illness or disease brings to the surface underlying family dynamics and issues. Each family member is going to have different opinions, thoughts, feelings, and coping mechanisms. Some will deny or ignore the problem, others will be positive and helpful, and some will tell you what you should be doing or what you're doing wrong. Some may stay away, and others may be physically unavailable due to distance.

Whatever your family dynamics, they can and will surface in times of hardship, such as dealing with your loved one's disease, and can make everything more frustrating and complicated for you. The bottom line is that family members are who they are. As much as you may want them to be different, they may not change. You can't control them. You can only control your expectations and your reactions to their behavior.

Generally, three scenarios occur when a family member has dementia:

- The caregiver spouse becomes disappointed with their children;
- The adult child caregiver is in conflict with siblings or other family members; and
- The caregiver spouse isn't receptive to getting assistance.

Caregiver Spouse Disappointed with Children

In the first scenario, the caregiver spouse takes care of the spouse with dementia. If the couple has children, the caregiver spouse may become disappointed if their children don't offer to help or stop by for visits. The caregiver spouse feels that the children are avoiding them, and they often ask themselves, "What did we do wrong?" Alternately, the adult children may be opinionated and critical of the caregiver spouse. Either way, the caregiver spouse may feel abandoned, judged, or unsupported by their children. This adds to the frustration that comes with being the primary caregiver.

One of the main reasons adult children stay away is that they're uncomfortable interacting with the parent who has dementia. For instance, they don't know what to talk about or what to do when they visit. Watching their parent decline is difficult and sad for some adult children. As a result, the children avoid the situation or distance themselves emotionally.

As frustrating as it can be to accept, each family member is coping to the best of their ability. Your time and energy are valuable. Try not to get caught up in attempting to force family members to change. Instead, find out what each family member is comfortable doing, and then find other resources to support you and your loved one with dementia.

> *Often, an illness or disease brings to the surface underlying family dynamics and issues.*

The first step in gathering an honest assessment of family members' contributions is to give each person an opportunity to express their concerns, feelings, thoughts, fears, and opinions about the disease and what they anticipate the care needs to be. This is beneficial for several reasons:

- It allows each family member to feel heard and understood.

- It allows everyone to express an interest in sharing responsibilities. This gives you a good idea of each family member's capacity and limitations so that you can plan accordingly.

- It allows you to share your fears, concerns, needs, and limitations so that they have realistic expectations of you.

- It gives everyone a chance to clear up misunderstandings.

If you decide to have a family meeting, consider having a third party — a family elder mediator, doctor, or a close family friend — facilitate the conversation among family members. You may not like everything you hear, but this process increases the chance that family members will be receptive to supporting and helping you. As difficult as this may be, try to accept each family member's limitations and focus on what they are willing to do or are capable of doing. This minimizes your frustration and disappointment.

Resentment builds up when people let us down. By having realistic expectations of family members, you can find other ways to fill the gaps so that you and your loved one get the support you need and deserve.

Adult Child as Caregiver

In the second scenario, an adult child takes care of a parent with dementia. Typically, one child is the primary caregiver. It can be challenging and frustrating when siblings or other family members don't offer to help, and even more so when they question your decisions or actions.

If your siblings challenge your decisions, remember that you are doing the best that you can. Let them know that you're reading and learning about the progression of dementia and that you're researching the best ways to deal with people living with dementia. Encourage your siblings to do the same. They may wish to read books about dementia, listen to podcasts, or meet with a dementia consultant. Once they become more educated, you can compare notes. Remind them that you're making choices with the intent of doing what is best for your parent — and sometimes, doing what is best for your parent is doing what is best for you.

Using the previous example of Kathy and her father, Kenneth, there comes the point when Kathy can't handle taking care of her father at home and wants to place him in an assisted living community. Kathy struggles with guilt but knows in her heart that she has reached her limits and can't take care of Kenneth at home.

Kathy desperately wants support from her two daughters, but she doesn't receive it. Instead, they tell Kathy that she is selfish and cruel to their grandfather. They ask, "How can you do this to Grandpa?"

Kathy agonizes over this decision. One day, she asks her daughters to spend two days at her house to visit with and care for their grandfather while she stays at a nearby hotel. One daughter stays for 24 hours and is completely exhausted by the time she returns home.

The other daughter lasts 12 hours and can't handle her grandfather's repetitive questioning, constant forgetfulness, and need for assistance with bathing and toileting. After learning firsthand how exhausting and challenging it is to take care of their grandfather at home, Kathy's daughters change their minds and support her decision to place Kenneth in a care community.

Until people walk in your shoes, they have no idea what you're dealing with. Therefore, you may need to make decisions that don't align with other family members' opinions. This doesn't mean that you're doing something wrong — it just means people express their views based on their limited understanding of dementia and their limited experience interacting or living with the person with dementia.

It's easy for other family members to challenge or criticize you, but remember, you're the person taking care of your loved one. You're the one living with them and taking care of them 24/7. And, if your loved one with dementia is not living with you, you're still the primary person visiting, checking in on them, and overseeing their care in the group living community. Other family members have limited experience dealing with the challenges you face. Their opinions are not based on your reality and hands-on experience.

It's crucial to set boundaries. If certain family members aren't willing to support your decisions, are constantly challenging you, or are difficult to deal with, you may have to reduce the amount of contact you have with them. You may want to inform difficult family members about your loved one's status by sending biweekly or monthly written progress reports. They'll stay in the loop and can't accuse you of keeping them in the dark. When you send updates, include both positive and negative changes or observations.

In extreme cases of armchair quarterbacking, you may have to completely cut off communication with a family member — at least temporarily. The same holds if a family member takes advantage of you or is abusive. If your loved one with dementia insists on seeing the family member who constantly challenges you, you may need to leave the premises or have a third party present so that you're not alone with that person. You may even need to insist on a supervised visit, where you aren't present but a neutral observer is.

You have to trust your reality and do what's in your best interest and what's in the best interest of your loved one with dementia. Unfortunately, this may involve making decisions about your loved one's care without the family support you would like. This doesn't mean your choices are wrong; it simply means they don't have your experience and perspective of the circumstances.

Caregiver Spouse is Resistant to Getting Help

In the third scenario, the caregiver spouse — the parent or significant other taking care of their spouse with dementia — isn't ready to admit that they need help. Using the previous example of Debra and DeShawn, Debra's daughter Susie witnesses DeShawn's struggle to take care of her mother and sees that her mother is declining. No matter what Susie says and does, she can't get DeShawn to do what is necessary to provide the proper care for Debra.

Rather than trying to convince her stepfather that he needs to hire more help, Susie learns that it's important to allow him to express his thoughts and feelings. She sets up a time to talk privately and give him a chance to share his concerns and fears and talk about why he won't accept help. This gives Susie insight into DeShawn's experience and his perception of the road ahead.

There are many reasons why a caregiver spouse may resist getting help. Typically, a combination of factors contributes to this mindset. They include:

Embarrassment. The caregiver spouse doesn't want the situation to reflect poorly on them, or they're trying to protect their spouse from being embarrassed by their behavior.

Denial. The caregiver spouse believes that they can manage everything and don't think additional support is needed. They don't see change as making things easier or better for them or their spouse. Often, the caregiver spouse goes to great lengths to cover up for the spouse with dementia. They downplay their loved one's symptoms and try to convince you that things are better than they are.

Guilt. The caregiver spouse experiences guilt about their relationship and feels it's their responsibility to take care of their loved one exclusively. They think they would be letting their loved one down if someone came into their home to help.

Failure. The caregiver spouse feels that they would be failing their loved one if they weren't the sole person taking care of them. They may perceive asking for help as an admission of failure, and they're afraid that their loved one with dementia will feel their spouse has given up on them.

Privacy. Many people have been raised to believe that what goes on behind closed doors stays behind closed doors. They refuse to accept help because they don't want strangers in their home or their privacy invaded.

Marriage Vows or Promises. The caregiver spouse doesn't want to break the marriage vows or promises the couple made to each other over the years. They feel obligated to fulfill their loved one's wishes and that accepting help is betraying their spouse.

Loss of Control. The caregiver spouse doesn't want to relinquish control. They are worried that others won't do things correctly, and the caregiver spouse doesn't want to be replaced.

What Ifs. The caregiver spouse is fearful of making things worse and worries about the "what ifs." What if the spouse with dementia gets angry or doesn't like someone coming into the home? What if the helper drops their loved one or doesn't know how to handle them? What if they or the spouse with dementia doesn't like the person who helps them?

Cost. The caregiver spouse either says they can't afford help or it's too expensive. Cost is usually a stated issue until the caregiver spouse sees the value and importance of having additional support.

Grief and Loss. In the mind of the caregiver spouse, accepting help forces them to admit to themselves that their loved one is declining and they aren't ready to deal with that sadness and loss. The type of loss the caregiver spouse experiences is called ambiguous loss, and the kind of grief they experience is called anticipatory grief.

From the caregiver spouse's point of view, these are valid reasons to resist getting help for themselves and the family member living with dementia.

Regardless of their rationale, avoid telling the caregiver spouse what you think they should be doing or that what they're doing is wrong — assuming that the spouse with dementia isn't being neglected or in danger. That will only alienate the caregiver spouse. It's important to give the caregiver spouse a chance to express their thoughts, feelings, concerns, and fears. This is essential to establishing an alliance with them.

Resistance occurs for a reason. It's a subconscious defense mechanism that gets triggered to protect us from emotions we're not ready to face. If the caregiver spouse is resistant to making changes, you need to embrace their resistance to break that resistance down. Here's how:

Listen to learn. The goal is to put aside your opinions and listen to their point of view without interrupting, correcting, or arguing with them. Listen as objectively as you can so that you fully understand their perspective. You may disagree with what they are saying, but you will better understand their issues and concerns when the conversation is over.

Ask leading questions. Encourage the caregiver spouse to talk about why they don't want to bring in help. You might say, "I want to understand your feelings and thoughts about why you don't want to bring in additional support to help you and Mom." Ask why they think they don't need help and ask about their concerns and fears. Determine the impact that getting help would have on them. For example, ask, "How do you think bringing in extra care will affect you and Mom?" and "If you did bring in outside care, what would you be comfortable with?"

Reminisce. Reminisce with the caregiver spouse. Tell stories and talk about memories. Bring up fun or funny experiences, and talk about your loved one's personality. This breaks down the caregiver spouse's defenses and establishes a positive connection between the two of you.

Substitute "support" for "help." Using the word "support" can be less threatening and more inviting. It may make the caregiver spouse feel that they are a part of the care team rather than being replaced or excluded. If the caregiver spouse feels they have a say in what is needed and how the support is provided, they may be more receptive to hiring additional care.

Validate. Write down the caregiver spouse's rationale for refusing additional support. Repeat and paraphrase what they tell you to make sure you hear them correctly and they feel listened to and understood. The goal is to understand their perspective without judgment or criticism.

List concrete indicators. Encourage the caregiver spouse to identify specific situations, behaviors, or red flags that indicate the need for more help, whether in the home or by placing their spouse in a care community. Examples of concrete indicators are when the spouse with dementia is:

- Experiencing urinary or bowel incontinence;
- No longer able to perform personal care activities like showering, dressing, toileting, or brushing their teeth;
- Refusing to accept help with personal hygiene;
- Exhibiting aggression or combative behaviors;
- Falling more frequently;
- Wandering;
- Shadowing;
- Exhibiting loss of appetite;

- Experiencing increased medical issues, such as urinary tract infections; or

- Getting up during the night or experiencing restless sleep.

Concrete indicators help justify the need for additional support, and they decrease the caregiver spouse's guilt or sense of failure. Indicators make the caregiver spouse more aware that the dementia has progressed and their loved one requires more care than they can provide on their own.

In addition, concrete indicators allow the caregiver spouse to see the value, importance, and need for additional care. They help the caregiver spouse accept reality in a way that is emotionally less threatening. It's a subtle way of breaking down the denial while keeping them in their comfort zone.

Avoid "shoulding" them. Avoid telling the caregiver spouse what you think they should be doing. This will immediately put them on the defensive. Instead, try to phrase your opinion as something you learned that you want to share with them. For example, you can say, "I was reading about wandering, and it was interesting that the article said that it's a good idea to put black mats in front of the exit doors." This style of communication is more educational and less judgmental. Afterward, you can have an open discussion about what you shared with them.

Be empathetic. The goal is to be able to relate to what the caregiver spouse is going through. You might say:

- "Help me understand your perspective."

- "I can't imagine how hard this is on you."

- "What do you think Mom needs right now?"
- "How can we lessen the stress or burden on you?"
- "Why do you feel you have to do this alone?"
- "At what point do you think caring for Mom might be too difficult to handle on your own?"
- "How is caring for Mom affecting you?"
- "How are you doing?"
- "What would make this easier on you?"
- "How do you feel when we suggest hiring additional care and support?"
- "What are your thoughts and concerns about hiring outside care?"
- "Do you think there will be a time when you may need to hire outside care?"
- "What kind of additional care would you be comfortable with?"

Your goal is to understand what the caregiver spouse is thinking and feeling. You want to know how caregiving is affecting them, as well as their fears and concerns. Once you figure out their reasons for not wanting to bring in additional care or support, you have a better idea of how to approach them.

Once the caregiver spouse feels that you're an ally, it increases the chance of working together to develop care options that are in everyone's best interest. Embracing the caregiver spouse's resistance is a skill that takes time, patience, and understanding, but it's well worth the effort.

Establishing an Emergency Plan

If you and your loved one with dementia are the only two people living in the home, it's essential to prepare for the unexpected and have an emergency plan in place. Trying to locate information and items while you're in crisis is next to impossible. You'll be better able to take care of your loved one if you take these steps before an emergency:

- Sign up for a life alert or medical alert program so that, if something happens to you, the appropriate authorities can be contacted on your behalf. When you sign up, make sure to let them know that your loved one has dementia, so they know what to expect when they arrive. If you are not living in your parents' house and the caregiver spouse isn't willing to sign up for a life alert or medical alert program, consider installing cameras in the home so that you can monitor what is happening at the house.

- There are seven legal and medical documents that you should complete and put into an easily accessible folder:

    1. **Living will.** Also known as an advance health care directive, a living will outlines your preferences about life-sustaining medical treatment if you are incapacitated and unable to make those decisions.

2. **Revocable living trust.** A revocable living trust allows you to control your finances and assets while you're alive and stipulates how you want your assets distributed upon your death.

3. **Financial power of attorney.** Financial power of attorney gives the person you designate the legal authority to make financial decisions on your behalf.

4. **Health care power of attorney.** Health care power of attorney gives the person you designate the legal authority to make health care decisions on your behalf if you are incapable of making decisions for yourself due to illness, injury, or incapacitation.

5. **Physician orders for life-sustaining treatment (POLST).** POLST is a bright pink medical order form signed by you and your doctor that specifies the medical treatment you want and do not want to receive during a serious illness or life-threatening situation.

6. **Do not resuscitate (DNR).** A doctor writes a do-not-resuscitate order and instructs health care providers to refrain from beginning cardiopulmonary resuscitation (CPR) if your heart stops beating or your breathing stops.

7. **Health Insurance Portability and Accountability Act (HIPAA) authorization form.** A HIPAA authorization form authorizes medical professionals to share your medical information with the individuals or organizations you designate.

- Make a list of doctors' names and phone numbers, as well as a list of the medications you and your loved one take. Place them in a labeled envelope on the refrigerator so they will be accessible to first responders.

- Make a list of passwords that you and your loved one use. Ensure it is readily available if you or a trusted person needs access to your online financial accounts or medical records.

- Post the name and phone number of a local contact person on the refrigerator so you can have someone physically present with you at the hospital.

Hiring In-Home Care

As dementia progresses, it becomes increasingly difficult to manage your loved one's care by yourself. At some point, you realize that you need to provide additional care — whether it's in-home care or placing your loved one in a care community. Either way, it's essential to plan for this eventuality.

Some people prefer to start with in-home support services and then move their loved one into a care community as their needs increase. Others prefer to move their loved one directly into a care community when they feel their home environment is no longer safe or they're unable to manage at-home care. There are no right or wrong answers. It comes down to:

- Your comfort level and capacity for caregiving;
- Your physical and emotional well-being;
- Your and your loved one's safety;

- The amount and type of care your loved one needs; and
- What is financially feasible.

Try not to wait for a crisis to occur before making a decision. Remember that you're making this decision to provide the best care for your loved one. It's an extension of your love, compassion, devotion, and commitment.

Deciding to hire in-home care can be stressful and overwhelming. It means admitting to yourself that your loved one needs more support than you can provide. In addition, hiring, coordinating, and navigating the type and amount of care your loved one needs is a big responsibility. But, once everything is in place, it gives you a break from day-to-day caregiving, allowing you to conserve your energy and spend more quality time with your loved one.

It can be difficult to know at what point you should reach out for in-home support. To start, ask yourself the following questions about your capacity for caregiving:

- Is it becoming more difficult to maintain your or your loved one's home?
- Is it becoming more difficult to manage your or your loved one's finances?
- Are you feeling increasingly overwhelmed, isolated, depressed, or frustrated?
- Is caring for your loved one taking a toll on your physical, mental, and emotional health?
- Are you feeling unmotivated to get out of bed?

- Is your sleep being interrupted?
- Are you sleep-deprived or exhausted?
- Are you or your loved one at a higher risk of getting hurt or falling?
- Are you having difficulty maintaining the quality of care your loved one needs?
- Are you having difficulty engaging your loved one in activities?
- Is it increasingly difficult to take your loved one on outings, such as to the grocery store or appointments?
- Are you having difficulty attending to your loved one's physical and cognitive needs?
- Is it becoming more challenging to maintain your loved one's hygiene and toileting habits?

Next, ask yourself the following questions about your loved one's needs:

- Is their health declining?
- Are they falling more frequently?
- Do they sleep a lot during the day?
- Are they refusing to leave the house?
- Are they withdrawing from participating in social activities?
- Are they bored, pacing, or agitated throughout the day?
- Are their household bills building up?

- Does their house look uncharacteristically disorganized or messy?
- Are they eating less or losing a significant amount of weight?
- Are they neglecting their hygiene?
- Are they having frequent urinary or bowel accidents?
- Have their driving skills declined?
- Are they missing scheduled appointments?
- Do they forget to take their medication?
- Do they cry frequently?

If you answered "yes" to several of these questions, it's an excellent time to consider bringing in outside support and care.

Understanding the in-home care process can help you navigate care options. The first step is knowing whether your loved one needs support with activities of daily living or if they also need some level of medical help.

If your loved one needs help with day-to-day living, you are looking for non-medical in-home care. This type of support can be described in many ways, including companion care, personal care, and non-medical care. These professionals typically help with:

- Companionship;
- Transportation to appointments;
- Running errands;
- Coordinating meal planning and cooking;

- Performing light housekeeping tasks and pet care;
- Assisting your loved one with eating and dressing;
- Engaging your loved one in activities;
- Help with personal hygiene tasks, such as bathing, toileting, and incontinence;
- Mobility and transfers; and
- Medication reminders.

If your family member needs a degree of medical support, you are looking for home health care that must be prescribed by a medical professional. Home health care is often needed after a hospitalization or surgery and allows skilled nursing or rehabilitation to be administered at home temporarily. In addition, home health professionals can teach primary caregivers how to perform some medical tasks, such as peritoneal dialysis; changing, cleaning, or emptying colostomy bags; and giving injections.

Your loved one's insurance may cover home health care services; if so, your loved one may need a prescription or referral from their primary care physician. Home health care can be administered by different types of health care professionals, including home health aides, nurses, and therapists.

The type of medical care provided by home health care professionals can include:

- Conducting speech, occupational, or physical therapy;
- Administering IV medication or injections;
- Providing wound care;

- Tracking vital signs and blood glucose levels;

- Pain and medication management;

- Changing, detaching, and attaching catheters and colostomy bags; and

- Monitoring the status of a serious illness or an unstable health condition to prevent complications or hospital readmission.

There are situations in which in-home care and home health care may be used simultaneously. Once you determine the type of care you need, make a list of your priorities. For example, when DeShawn realizes that he needs non-medical in-home care for his wife, Debra, he makes the following list:

- **Dependable.** Caregivers arrive when they say they will arrive, are on time, and don't leave before the end of their shift.

- **Consistent.** Caregivers have an established weekly schedule, so the days and times are the same each week. Two weeks' notice is provided if a caregiver is taking time off.

- **No revolving door.** Turnover remains low among caregivers. The same one or two individuals regularly come instead of having five or six people coming in and out of the house.

- **Cognitive stimulation.** Caregivers provide activities that engage and stimulate Debra.

- **Physical stimulation.** Caregivers take Debra out for walks, do gentle exercises, and take her on outings.

- **Personal care.** Caregivers assist with personal hygiene, showering, dressing, and toileting.
- **Companionship.** Caregivers provide socialization and emotional support.
- **Meal planning.** Caregivers provide help with meal preparation and cooking.
- **Focused attention.** Caregivers aren't on their cell phones and don't watch TV.

Having this type of list ahead of time helps you outline your needs and allows you to set expectations with your chosen care team.

You can begin the process of hiring in-home care by asking for referrals from family members, friends, doctors, elder care professionals, local senior centers, community organizations, your Area Agency on Aging, or faith-based organizations. Once you have recommendations, you can gather more information during the screening process.

When you speak with in-home care agencies, it's a good idea to ask a broad range of questions centered on your loved one's unique needs, as well as:

- **Is the care agency licensed by the state?** Most in-home care and home health agencies require licensure. Research your state's licensing requirements before making a final decision.
- **Are caregivers bonded?** If a caregiver steals, agency bonding gives you the right to file a claim up to the bond amount.

- **Do caregivers have workers' compensation coverage?** Whether they are employees or contractors, caregivers should have workers' compensation coverage. It provides you with liability protection if a caregiver is injured while working for your family. Identifying the responsible party in an emergency is especially important with private caregivers.

- **How long has the home care agency been in business?** A minimum of two years in business demonstrates that the agency is stable.

- **Is the home care agency privately owned or a franchise?** If the agency is privately owned, speak to the owner and ask what inspired them to start a care agency. A franchise typically has standardized policies and procedures, while a privately-owned home care agency may have more flexibility in its policies and procedures. Whether privately owned or a franchise, you're looking for a home care agency that can provide the best quality of care and accommodate your loved one's needs.

- **What is the agency's screening process for caregivers?** At a minimum, they should conduct a background check, contact references, and confirm prior caregiver experience. Ask how many personal and professional references are required when a caregiver applies for a job and what experience the agency looks for when hiring a caregiver.

- **Do they subject caregivers to background checks and drug screenings?** You want to make sure the people working for you have been thoroughly screened.

- **What kind of and how often is dementia training provided to caregivers?** Dementia care requires a specific skill set and level of expertise. Make sure the caregivers have dementia-specific training or experience. In-person or online training should be provided by a dementia consultant, educator, or specialist and should be conducted at least every six months for a minimum of three hours.

- **How are caregivers monitored and supervised?** Caregivers should report to a supervisor or case manager regularly to ensure the quality of care, monitor the needs of your loved one, and update the care plan as necessary.

- **Do they charge you for a weekly minimum number of hours?** Most agencies have a minimum number of hours per shift or week, but this varies depending on the agency.

- **Are they willing to work with you if you can't meet the minimum requirements initially but the goal is to work up to the minimum requirements?** Some agencies are willing to negotiate this as long as the intent is gradually increasing the hours to meet their minimum requirements.

- **Do they provide service 24 hours a day, 7 days a week?** There must be someone you can contact 7 days a week at any time of day or night.

- **What kind of staff do they employ?** They may employ caregivers, registered nurses, care managers, physical therapists, speech therapists, or occupational therapists. In-home care agencies employ caregivers and case managers with professional or personal caregiving experience. Home health care agencies hire medical professionals, such as registered nurses and therapists.

- **Who will do the initial assessment of your loved one?** Usually, a supervisor or case manager does the assessment for in-home care. A medical professional does the evaluation if you're hiring home health care.

- **Do they have restrictions, such as weight restrictions or medication administration restrictions?** In-home care agencies are not allowed to administer medication, but they can provide medication reminders. Home health care dispenses and administers medication directly to the patient. Some agencies impose weight restrictions to avoid bringing in additional equipment or a second staff member to move your loved one.

- **What is their cancellation policy?** This varies from agency to agency, but most require at least 48 hours' notice.

- **Who do you speak to if you're dissatisfied with a caregiver?** Typically, you talk to the supervisor, case manager, care manager, or agency owner.

- **Are there additional fees?** Usually, an agency charges extra fees for federal holidays and overtime, but this varies from agency to agency.

- **Do they provide a backup caregiver? If so, what is the timeframe for finding a backup?** They should provide a backup caregiver as soon as possible, but it often depends on the availability of additional staff.

- **Do they accept long-term care insurance for in-home care or health insurance for home health care?** Are there other benefits for which you could apply? Most in-home care agencies are private pay but do accept long-term care insurance or VetAssist. Check with the home care agency and your long-term care insurance provider to determine what services are covered and how payments are made. Home health care is often covered by Medicare, Medicaid, or Medicaid waiver programs; private health insurance; or private pay.

Before ending your conversation, ask the agency to send you written material that outlines the services they provide and the fees they charge. This allows you to read and discuss the information before making a final decision. It can also be helpful to read online reviews because they can identify other questions to ask.

You can also choose to hire private in-home caregivers. If you go this route, keep in mind that you are becoming an employer. For example, you need to conduct a criminal background and reference check, negotiate rates, and pay payroll taxes. You may need to obtain additional insurance to cover liability, bonding, and workers' compensation. You are also responsible for finding a replacement caregiver if the person isn't able to work a scheduled shift.

Questions to ask when you meet a private in-home caregiver:

- Have they worked with people with dementia? How many? How often?

- What do they like the most about working with people with dementia?

- What is the biggest challenge they encounter when working with someone with dementia? How do they deal with this?

- What dementia training have they had?

- What made them want to become a caregiver?

- How long have they been a caregiver?

- Do they have professional liability insurance?

Hiring in-home care provides you with more time for yourself, takes the pressure off of you to be "on" all of the time, reduces your stress and burnout, and frees you up to be your loved one's partner, daughter, or son and not only their "caregiver." Often, families find that their loved one is more cooperative and responsive to an agency or private caregiver than they are to a family caregiver.

At some point, as dementia progresses and your loved one's needs increase, you will face the decision to either extend care at home or move your loved one into a care community.

Suppose you decide to extend care at home, possibly providing 24-hour care. In that case, it's comforting to know that a caregiver is available to offer emotional support, reduce the risk of falling, and provide assistance with daily living activities.

Placement

Sherry and Stanley have always been the envy of their friends. Their 50-year marriage began with a storybook romance, and they've been best friends and lovers ever since. They always shared their innermost thoughts and deepest desires with one another and often talked about their later years. Sherry often told Stanley that she never wanted to be kept alive without fully living and that the worst outcome she could imagine was being put in "one of those places." Once Sherry was diagnosed with dementia, her decline was rapid, and Stanley wrestled with his promise to her and the reality that he could no longer care for her at home.

Deciding whether or not to place your loved one in a care community can be an excruciating decision. It's common to ask:

- When is the right time to move my loved one to a care community?
- Is placing my loved one in a care community the only option?
- Why can't I manage to care for my loved one at home?
- What can I afford?
- How am I going to pay for my loved one's care?

Like Stanley, caregivers often feel guilty, feel like failures, or feel that they're letting their loved one down when they're no longer able to care for them at home. This is reinforced if they've had discussions or made promises to their loved one before their dementia diagnosis.

The truth is that, in many cases, dementia doesn't allow you to take care of your loved one at home. The demands, challenges, and responsibilities simply become too difficult to manage on your own. It's worth repeating that *dementia* doesn't allow you to take care of your loved one at home. Dementia is responsible for putting you in this position.

You have not failed. You are not letting your loved one down. You are demonstrating your love and support by providing the care that they need. There will come a time when you won't be able to do everything by yourself, and placement may be a necessity. Placement is not just for the health and well-being of your loved one, but also for your financial, physical, mental, and emotional well-being.

People with dementia have unique needs, and a dementia care community is designed to meet those needs. There is an entire staff trained in dementia care that is looking after your loved one. In addition to memory loss, dementia symptoms can include delusions, agitation, extreme personality changes, hallucinations, confusion, incontinence, and disorientation — all of which are very difficult to manage on your own. Often, dementia requires specialized care from professionals trained to meet the various challenges of people living with the disease.

Unfortunately, many families put off making this difficult decision until their loved one experiences a health crisis. It's essential to have a plan in place so that you're not rushed into a decision while feeling pressured and unprepared.

Even though Stanley was heartbroken about the idea of placing Sherry in a care community, he had access to the following list of questions. His answers helped Stanley assess Sherry's needs as her disease progressed and prepared him to make the decision to place her.

> *One of the most difficult decisions a caregiver has to make is placing your loved one in a care community. This can be an excruciating decision.*

As your loved one's needs change, ask yourself questions about various aspects of your and your loved one's lives.

Their Physical Health and Safety

- Is your loved one wandering? Are they getting out of the house without you realizing it? Are they having difficulty finding their way back home?

- Is your loved one safe living at home? For example, does a lack of balance put them at higher risk of falling, or are they disoriented and confused about where they are?

- Does your loved one have recurring infections, such as urinary tract infections?

- Is medication management a challenge? Are they refusing to take their medication, or is it difficult to coordinate their medication schedule?

- Do they have mobility issues? Are they falling more frequently, unstable on their feet, or having difficulty getting out of a chair?

- Is their health declining? Has their diabetes, hypertension, heart disease, stenosis, or wound worsened?

- Is their appetite decreasing? Are they refusing to eat? Are they losing weight?
- Are they experiencing increased difficulty swallowing or controlling their bowels and bladder?
- Are they sleep-deprived?

Your Physical Health and Safety

- Is your physical health negatively impacted by taking care of your loved one? Are you experiencing heart palpitations, high blood pressure, uncontrolled diabetes, rashes, twitches, headaches, stomachaches, or sleep deprivation?
- If your loved one falls, are you able to help them up without hurting yourself?
- Has your hygiene suffered? Are you not bathing, brushing your teeth, or doing laundry as frequently as you used to?
- Is your loved one physically aggressive, or do they have violent outbursts?

Their Behavior and Mental Health

- Is your loved one's behavior becoming challenging to handle?
- Are they becoming increasingly frustrated, agitated, angry, or hostile?
- Are they crying or saying that they want to die?
- Does your loved one anxiously pace?

- Have they lost all interest in people, places, and things they once enjoyed?
- Is your loved one isolated, lacking in social interaction, or refusing to engage in activities?
- Do they need help starting an activity they were once able to do easily on their own?

Your Mental Health

- Are you frequently angry, irritable, or agitated?
- Do you frequently cry?
- Is it becoming increasingly difficult for you to get out of bed to care for your loved one?
- Do you worry about your safety or their safety?
- Are you able to maintain your home, health, finances, relationships, social activities, hobbies, and professional work?
- Do you feel pulled in a million different directions trying to juggle your own family, your work, and your parents' care?

Limitations of Care

- Is it becoming increasingly difficult to care for your loved one's hygiene? Are they refusing to bathe, brush their teeth, or change their clothes?
- Are you able to provide the ongoing cognitive and physical stimulation your loved one needs?

- Is your loved one incontinent or having daily toileting accidents?
- Do you have to make an increasing number of home modifications — for example, grab bars or ramps — to manage your loved one's needs?

If you answer "yes" to many of these questions, it may be time for you to consider moving your loved one into a care community. Selecting where to place your loved one depends upon their needs, interests, preferences, and how much the disease has progressed.

Before visiting care communities, prioritize the accommodations and services that are important to you. You may want to consider these factors:

Physical Facility

Location. What is the farthest distance you want to travel?

Environment. Do you prefer light vs. dark spaces? Do you want an open and airy floor plan or a closed and hotel-like atmosphere? Is it important that there are common areas outdoors?

Cleanliness. Is there an odor when you visit? Are the rooms and carpets clean? Is there dust? Are the trash cans full?

Rooms. Are there private rooms? What are the different sizes of rooms? How do they determine how to pair residents in semi-private rooms?

Hospice. How many hospice beds do they provide for end-of-life care? Which hospice services do they use?

Staffing

Staffing Ratio. What is the ratio of staff to patients? Ideally, you're looking for a 6:1 resident-to-staff ratio or better. However, the staffing ratio depends on the number of residents and those residents' individual care needs.

Staff Composition. Are there RNs, LVNs or LPNs, and MDs on staff, and do they work onsite or remotely?

Staff Training. Do they provide dementia training for the staff? If so, what are the training requirements? Who provides the training?

Medical Care

Medical. What medical services do they provide? What do they do when an emergency occurs? What do they consider an emergency? What is the policy for a medical or ER visit? Can a resident come back if they have to go to rehab after a hospital stay?

Medication Management. What is their medication management protocol? What is the protocol when a doctor changes your loved one's medication? Who is responsible for picking up medications?

Financial Factors

Financial. Is it affordable? What are the costs for private rooms and semi-private rooms?

Policies and Fees. What does the monthly payment include? What is not included in the monthly fee?

Resident Care

Resident Criteria. What criteria does the person living with dementia have to meet to be a resident in their community? What would get a resident evicted from the community?

Types of Care. What kinds of care do they provide? What kinds of care do they not offer? Can your loved one live there until end-of-life? What happens when they are no longer ambulatory? Do they provide care for all levels of activities of daily living?

Safety and Security. How close is the nearest hospital and fire station? What security systems do they have in place? What are their emergency and disaster plans?

Outside Care. Can you supplement your loved one's care by hiring additional support from outside the care community? Under what circumstances would you be required to hire outside care services for your loved one?

Outings. How often do they take residents on outings? Is there a separate charge for outings? How do they deal with a resident who doesn't want to participate in the activities? Do they have companion care services? Are companion care services an additional fee?

Stimulation. Ask for a month's worth of daily activity schedules. What kinds of activities do they offer, and when do they offer them? Are there enough activities that your loved one enjoys?

What you're looking for in a care community depends upon your loved one's needs. It's important to tour multiple care communities to make an informed decision. Keep in mind that you're looking for the "right fit" for your loved one, so prioritize the factors that are most important for you. For example, Stanley decided that these factors were the most important for Sherry's care:

- Enclosed walking and outdoor common areas;
- Physical and cognitive activities;
- Social stimulation;
- Tasks that make her feel special;
- Having a room near the dining hall;
- Care community supplies her adult underwear and pads;
- The interior of the care community is well lit;
- The community is within a ten-mile radius of their home;
- Three meals per day are provided and included in the cost;
- Attentive and friendly staff.

When touring a care community, the most important questions to ask yourself are: How do you feel when touring the community? What is your first impression? What is your gut reaction? Trust your instincts.

Transitioning into a Care Community

Deciding to place your loved one in a care community can be difficult and heartbreaking. Once you've made that decision, the next challenge is approaching them and dealing with the aftermath of the move.

These eight steps will help you through this process:

Step 1: Deciding what to tell your loved one and how to approach them. There's no single right way to communicate with your loved one. In some instances, you can be honest, and your loved one accepts this decision. But if you think your loved one won't accept the truth or understand the need for a care community, it may be better to make up a story or embellish the truth. A compassionate lie, also known as a therapeutic act of kindness, may be in their best interest because it aims to minimize potential emotional distress.

Alternatively, you may want to consider speaking to your loved one's physician or an elder care professional and let them talk to your loved one about moving into a care community. This prevents you from becoming the bad guy.

These are examples of the stories that family caregivers have told their loved ones when moving them into a care community:

- "I have to go out of town to take care of Henry, and you won't be able to come with me. While I'm gone, you get to stay at a B&B. We'll both be staying somewhere special."
- "The doctor wants your diabetes monitored. You're going to stay at a place that can help get it stabilized."
- "The house is being treated for termites, and we can't stay here. I'm going to stay at Mary's, and I've found somewhere nice for you to stay."
- "I'm having minor surgery and need time to recover. I won't be able to take care of you, so you're going to stay someplace nice until I get better."
- "The doctor wants you to go to rehab so you can get stronger."

- "My knee is bothering me, and the doctor wants me to go to rehab to make it stronger. While I'm in rehab, I found a nice place for you to stay. I will see you soon."

Deciding how far in advance to tell your loved one that they are moving depends on how you think they will react and how far the disease has advanced. If you tell them too early, you risk the possibility of causing anticipation anxiety, which can trigger an extremely negative reaction. If you think your loved one will react negatively, it may be best to wait as long as possible.

Regardless of when you tell your loved one, avoid telling them they are moving because they need more help. Typically, people living with dementia don't think they need help, especially if they cannot see their deficits. In addition, give your loved one the impression that the move is temporary. It's comforting and reassuring if they think the move isn't permanent.

> *'Don't be scared. Everyone here is very nice and you will meet lots of new friends!' My mom said these words to me when I went to kindergarten. This weekend I said these words to her as she started the next chapter of her life. We officially changed roles. I knew the day would come but it's still a shock. I find myself cheering for her to accept her 'new normal,' the way she cheered for me growing up!*
>
> — Debra Powers

Step 2: Setting up their room. The transition will be smoother if their room resembles their home bedroom. Bring their furniture, art, family photos, bedspread, sheets, and favorite items. Make sure to check with the care community about items that are prohibited. Often, live plants or flowers, cleaning products, and pictures in glass frames are not allowed.

Step 3: Coordinating the move. Before the day of the move, coordinate with other family members, the care community, and possibly your loved one's physician. Plan the logistics of the transition. Everyone needs to be on the same page as to the story, who will transport your loved one, who will greet them at the care community, and the best time to depart from the care community without your loved one. The goal is to have a thought-out plan, but sometimes, even the best-laid plans can encounter a glitch, so it's important to be flexible.

To help make the transition easier for the care community, share with them personal information about your loved one. For example, talk to the care community about your loved one's preferred activities, hobbies, prior career, likes and dislikes, food preferences or special dietary needs, daily routine, and morning and bedtime habits.

Once you've dropped off your loved one, the care community's goal is to engage your loved one in activities immediately. They will also try to pair your loved one with other residents that have something in common with your loved one.

Step 4: Check in with the care community. Call the care community to get an update as to how your loved one is adjusting. This information determines when you should visit them. The timeframe will vary depending on how well your loved one acclimates to their new environment. It could be anywhere between a few days to a couple of weeks. The goal is to have your loved one adjust to the community's routine (meal times, exercise, outings, and other activities) as soon as possible. This makes the transition smoother for your loved one and the care community.

Step 5: Prepare distractions in advance. When you visit, have a list of enjoyable topics or distractions ready so that you can redirect your loved one if they are angry or upset with you. If they are mad at you, don't extend your visit. Leave and try again another day. Ask the director of nursing, the assisted living coordinator, or the memory care coordinator when it might be best to visit again. Then, check with the care community in advance before your next visit.

Step 6: Prepare responses in advance. Anticipate how your loved one might react when they see you and formulate responses before your visit. As a result of dementia, they may say hurtful things. Seeing them angry and upset may tug at your heartstrings. Examples of what they may say include:

- "How could you do this to me?"
- "Why did you put me out to pasture?"
- "You're just trying to get rid of me."
- "Get me out of here!"
- "I don't belong here!"
- "I want to go home."
- "When can I go home?"
- "Why am I here?"
- "You just want all of my money."
- "You're having an affair and don't want me around."

- "Why did you dump me off?"
- "I was told you would do this to me."
- "What did I do wrong?"
- "I will be a good girl."
- "I don't deserve this."
- "I love you and want to be with you."

When you know that you're doing what is best for your loved one, these are painful things to hear. They can make you question if you made the right decision. You might even be tempted to bring them home. Hang in there. Your loved one will eventually adjust to their new environment. You did the right thing.

To help you get through this challenging time, respond to your loved one compassionately and empathetically. Here are some validating responses you can use:

- "Thank you for letting me know you're angry and upset with me. I apologize, and I love you."
- "I'm sorry you feel [repeat the same words they use]. I brought your favorite candy. Would you like some?"
- "Thank you for bringing this to my attention. I'm sorry you're upset. I remember the time when we [describe a trip or a fun time]."
- "Thank you for letting me know how you feel. I love you, and it's so good to see you."

- "I don't know when you can go home, but I will look into it. I love you."
- "I will give them your phone number so you can talk to them."
- "I will call them for you and let them know where you are."
- "I'm sorry. I love you very much."

Once you validate what your loved one is saying and provide a comforting response, immediately redirect your loved one's attention. Bring up a topic or begin an activity that interests them or makes them happy. For example, hand them a favorite food, read their favorite poem, watch TV, or pull out a deck of playing cards. The goal is to acknowledge how they feel and then move on so their brain becomes engaged in a pleasurable activity or topic.

If your loved one has a positive reaction when you see them, you can say something like:

- "It's so good to see you."
- "I've been looking forward to seeing you."
- "I enjoy spending time with you."
- "I'm enjoying our time together."
- "I brought something you like."
- "I love you."
- "I'm thinking about you."

If your loved one complains that people are mean to them or don't like them or that they aren't being fed, simply say you will look into it. Then, check with the director or manager to determine how things are going and tell them what your loved one is saying. Keep in mind that your loved one has dementia and could be distorting reality.

When you visit, focus on being happy to see your loved one. Try not to argue, explain, correct them, or make promises. Avoid mentioning home or how lonely you are, and don't expect them to remember something you previously told them. Keep the visit positive and focused on your loved one.

Step 7: Length of visit. How long to visit varies from person to person. It often depends on how well your loved one has settled in and if they're happy to see you. Check with the care community and ask for their advice for an appropriate length of time. Usually, 30 minutes is reasonable if you're not eating a meal with them. If you're staying for a meal, then the length of time may be extended.

The best times to visit are usually in the late morning before lunch, at lunchtime if you want to dine together, or in the early afternoon right after lunch. It's best to know when meals are scheduled so that you can plan your arrival time accordingly. It's also a good idea to let the care community know that you are coming to visit.

Step 8: Get emotional support. This transition can be more difficult for the primary caregiver and the family than for the person living with dementia. After all, you're also going through an adjustment period. Moving your loved one reinforces the reality that they are declining. You may be living alone for the first time and miss them terribly. Or you may be relieved and feel guilty about your relief. Get support by talking about your feelings, concerns, and fears with family members and friends or a counselor, religious leader, or support group.

Remember that your loved one will eventually adjust to living in their new environment — and so will you. It can take longer for some people than for others. Be patient with yourself and give yourself time to adjust to this profound change in your life.

Not only will your loved one settle in, but they may even thrive because they have more cognitive and physical stimulation, social interactions, structure to their day, emotional support, and independence. Love them. Support them in their new environment. Continue to be their advocate. And, know that you are doing a fantastic job taking care of them every step of the way.

Hospice Care

You may want to consider hospice care in the end stage of dementia, when your loved one has six months or less to live and the disease continues to progress. Hospice care focuses on your loved one's quality of life and not on treating or curing the disease. The goal of hospice care is to keep your loved one as comfortable as possible throughout the last phase of their life.

As your loved one's caregiver, it's essential to be able to recognize the signs of end-stage dementia, which include:

- Being bedridden and requiring 24-hour care;
- Being unable to speak or speaking gibberish;
- Needing help with eating and self-care;

- Loss of appetite or weight loss;
- Dehydration due to difficulty drinking and swallowing;
- Inability to walk or sit up without assistance;
- Contractures in the leg, arm, or hand that are difficult to straighten;
- Increased vulnerability to a variety of infections, including pneumonia, UTIs, and even sepsis;
- Hospitalizations and emergency room visits;
- Bowel or urinary incontinence; and
- Diagnosis of other medical conditions, such as cancer, kidney disease, congestive heart failure, or chronic obstructive pulmonary disease.

Hospice care focuses on four primary areas:

1. Medical care in the form of pain and symptom management;
2. Emotional and spiritual support for the patient and family members;
3. Respite care for the family caregiver; and
4. Grief and bereavement counseling.

An authorization from your loved one's doctor can initiate hospice care, or you can contact a hospice care provider directly. Once the wheels are set in motion, a team of hospice professionals meets with you and your loved one's doctor to create a care plan. Hospice can be provided wherever your loved one lives. Most hospice care is provided in the home, but it can also be provided in hospitals, nursing homes, care communities, and hospice facilities. Hospice care is typically covered by Medicare, Medicaid, and private insurance.

Once your loved one is in hospice care, you have around-the-clock access to your hospice team. The team typically includes:

- A physician that oversees medical care needs and prescribes medications;

- A nurse that can make medication adjustments, modify care plans, and identify the signs of dying;

- A home health aide that can assist with personal care and hygiene;

- A social worker that can provide professional and community resources for the family and patient;

- A counselor or chaplain that can provide counseling and bereavement support; and

- Volunteers that can help with household chores, errands, and companion care.

Before selecting a hospice agency, ask for referrals from family members, friends, doctors, elder care professionals, local senior centers, community organizations, your Area Agency on Aging, or faith-based organizations. Once you have recommendations, you can gather more information during the screening process.

When you speak with hospice agencies, ask:

- **How long has the hospice agency been in business?** Two years or more provides a track record. Ask for references and look up online reviews.

- **Who owns the hospice agency, and what is their background?** Look for experience in end-of-life care.

- **What services does the hospice agency provide?** It should provide a medical director; nurse care manager and nurses; social workers; spiritual, mental health, or bereavement counseling; dietary counseling; home health aides; medications; medical equipment; respite care; family education and support; and volunteers. If appropriate, hospice might provide physical, occupational, speech, and music therapists; and laboratory or diagnostic tests.

- **What services does the hospice agency provide to keep your loved one comfortable?** It should provide compassionate care, pain management, non-pain symptom control, medications, medical supplies, medical equipment, personal care, and psychological and spiritual support. The goal of hospice care is to provide comfort, relieve pain, and promote quality of life until the end of life.

- **How often does a nurse or other hospice staff visit?** It's typical for staff to visit between one and three times per week, depending on the patient's condition.

- **Will there be a single nurse or care manager overseeing your loved one's care?** A single nurse or care manager is important, as they can provide continuity of care.

- **How long does it take for the on-call nurse to arrive?** The on-call nurse should arrive within 30 to 45 minutes. Alternately, ask what would be the longest it would take the on-call nurse to arrive. Most on-call nurses travel long distances, so you want to have a realistic idea about when to expect their arrival.

- **Is the hospice agency accredited by The Joint Commission, Accreditation Commission for Health Care, or another accreditation body?** Accreditation means that the agency has met or exceeded the standards of the accreditation body.

- **Does the agency have 24-hour on-call access 7 days a week?** They should have around-the-clock, on-call access.

- **What is the hospice agency's experience providing care for people with dementia?** It's beneficial to hire a hospice agency experienced in caring for patients with dementia, and that provides regular dementia training to staff so that the care team knows how to support patients with dementia.

- **Are they Medicare-certified?** Costs are lower if your loved one receives Medicare and the agency is Medicare-certified.

- **Can you change hospice agencies if you're not satisfied with the care?** Make sure to ask about their cancellation policy. For example, the agency might require a 30-day notice in writing.

Hospice can be a very positive experience for you as a caregiver and for your loved one. Sometimes, a patient can improve as a result of the extra care they receive from hospice. For example, they may start eating more and gaining weight. If at some point it looks like your loved one will live longer than six months, hospice may be terminated. However, they can qualify for hospice care again as their health declines.

Your loved one will likely die of a medical complication related to their underlying dementia. For example, Debra dies from aspiration pneumonia, which occurs due to swallowing difficulties. Kathy's father, Kenneth, dies from a blood clot in his lung due to being immobile. Sometimes, the cause of death listed on a death certificate will say end-stage dementia because dementia is a terminal illness.

When the time comes, and your loved one isn't able to communicate or respond to you, it's still possible to connect with them by:

- Holding hands;
- Playing their favorite music;
- Telling them "I love you," "I'm thinking of you," and "I miss you;"
- Reading a prayer, quote, or story that has personal meaning and significance;
- Rubbing lotion on their skin;
- Brushing their hair; and
- Looking at old photos.

It's essential to tell the hospice team how you would like to spend time with your loved one during their final days and hours. Tell them whether or not you want to be with your loved one when they die, and how you would like to say goodbye.

Bereavement

After your loved one passes, you may experience conflicting feelings and emotions. On the one hand, you may feel relieved that this journey is finally over. On the other hand, you may feel guilty that you feel relieved. And, at the same time, you're mourning the loss of your loved one.

The bereavement process begins after your loved one passes away. How you grieve depends on your beliefs, faith, life experiences, and the type of loss you've suffered. And, there is no finite time in which you should finish dealing with your loss. Grieving is an individual process.

During this time, your feelings and emotions may fluctuate. Sadness is often the primary feeling most people associate with bereavement, but other important feelings and emotions are also normal. These include feeling:

- Loss and the finality of not having your loved one in your life;
- Relief that your loved one isn't suffering;
- Anger at the disease or what you've been through;
- Uncertainty about your future;
- Guilt that stems from questioning and reflecting on your past caregiving decisions;
- Acceptance that the journey is over and you can move on with your life;

- Free from the demands and responsibilities of taking care of your loved one;
- Anxious or worried about what your future without your loved one will be like;
- Depressed about how dementia impacted your life with your loved one;
- Nostalgic about the past;
- Anticipation about spending more time with family and friends;
- Afraid of living alone;
- Grateful that you aren't responsible for your loved one's care or making major decisions on their behalf;
- Numb, as though you're walking around in a daze or fog;
- Pain or emptiness that there's a hole in your life;
- Unable to accept what you've been through;
- Isolated and alone;
- Lost, questioning your purpose in life;
- Shock, even though you expected your loved one to die;
- A struggle with being a widow or widower, or losing a parent;
- Overwhelmed with paperwork; and
- Freedom in being able to move on with your life.

Whatever you're feeling is okay. Try not to judge or criticize yourself. Instead, work toward accepting that this is part of the grieving process. Have self-compassion and freely experience your feelings and emotions. Try not to compare your grief with that of other people. No two people are exactly alike, and no two people grieve exactly the same way.

Each person's bereavement process is unique. You may want to talk to family members and friends more often in order to share your grief. You may find comfort in joining a support group created to help people through the grieving process. You may even find that you don't immediately grieve after your loved one passes.

Sometimes, it can take months or years for feelings to surface. This delayed grief can occur when you least expect it and is more likely to occur if:

- You cared for a loved one for an extended period;
- You're not ready to deal with your feelings and emotions; or
- You're constantly busy doing practical tasks.

Similarly, each person is affected differently by the passing of a loved one. Sometimes, it can be difficult to adjust to living without them. Others more readily accept what has happened and are ready to move on. It's hard to be objective about your bereavement process, which is why it's a good idea to postpone making major financial and other life decisions.

Days, weeks, or months after your loss, you may find comfort and feelings of connection in:

- Giving yourself time to contemplate your loss while not cutting yourself off from other people;
- Embracing the moments you think you see or hear your loved one's voice;
- Displaying objects that were meaningful to your loved one, such as their favorite hat, bracelet, or quilt;
- Writing a letter to your loved one;
- Planting a bush or tree in your loved one's memory;
- Contributing to your loved one's favorite organization or charity;
- Making a weekly, monthly, or yearly visit to the cemetery where they are buried;
- Scattering their ashes outdoors by sea, air, or land;
- Compiling a photo album of their life and times;
- Writing your thoughts, feelings, and emotions in a journal;
- Creating a ritual by reading a poem, singing a song, or reciting a prayer daily, weekly, or monthly;
- Going to the ocean or taking hikes to be close to them;
- Cutting flowers and placing them on the counter, table, or desk where they sat or worked, or placing flowers near a photo of them;
- Asking for help from friends or family members if special events such as anniversaries, holidays, or birthdays are difficult;

- Honoring your spiritual needs by meditating, praying, carving out quiet time for reflection, singing songs, writing poems, or talking to a spiritual guide or leader;
- Looking for bereavement support groups and services if your grief seems insurmountable; or
- Seeking professional help if your grief is debilitating, preventing you from living, or if you feel suicidal.

You may consider starting an annual ritual in memory or as a celebration of your loved one's life. For example, those who practice Judaism have a tradition of lighting a candle the evening before their loved one's passing and letting it burn all day on the anniversary of their death. You might also consider cooking their favorite meal or going to their favorite restaurant on the anniversary of their passing. Or, visit the ocean or mountains and spread flower seeds in a celebration of their life.

Mourning the finality of your loss takes time, patience, support, and self-compassion. Give yourself time to accept your loss, process your thoughts and feelings, and adjust to living without your spouse, partner, parent, friend, or family member.

It's been a long journey filled with responsibilities and challenges, ups and downs, and difficult decisions. Be patient, loving, and gentle with yourself. Ask for support as you work through this time of your life. Above all, give yourself permission to move on with your own life.

Action Plan: Paving the Way

1. Adapting to your loved one's changes involves increasing your awareness and understanding of potential triggers. Put on your investigative hat and begin using the Observational Log and Caregiver Trigger Log found in the Appendix.

2. While each dementia journey is unique, planning can make the journey easier. If you don't have an emergency plan, now's a great time to create one.

3. Become acquainted with in-home care agencies, tour care communities, or inquire about hospice care if the disease is progressing and you or your loved one need additional support.

Part III

The 4 D's of Dementia Care

As dementia progresses, it becomes increasingly difficult to get your loved one to act in ways that support their well-being, such as bathing, toileting, brushing their teeth, and changing their clothes. Your initial approach may be to try and use logic to reason with them. Reasoning and logic usually don't work and often can make the situation worse.

Instead, replace logic and reasoning with the 4 D's of Dementia Care: detach, document, diffuse, and distract. While easier said than done, these four steps will help you manage your caregiver journey. Don't expect perfection when implementing these strategies. They require patience and practice, as well as trial and error. Treat yourself with love and kindness as you explore these techniques.

Detach: Don't take it personally. Remind yourself that your loved one doesn't have control over what they say and do. Dementia is to blame. This reminder allows you to be more objective about your loved one's behaviors.

Document: Write down your observations when your loved one's mood changes or when their behavior becomes difficult. The intent is to uncover any patterns or triggers. If you can figure out the causes, you'll have a better chance of solving the problem or minimizing the frequency and intensity of the behavior.

Diffuse: Acknowledge their feelings, validate what they are saying using their exact words, and reassure them that they are safe and that things will be okay. Your empathy can have a calming effect and helps you better understand their underlying concerns.

Distract: Redirect their attention by encouraging them to focus on an activity they enjoy or changing the topic to one that engages them. Redirecting can decrease your loved one's distress and keep the behavior from spiraling out of control.

Caregiving can be lonely. It can feel like you're the only one dealing with the difficult behaviors caused by dementia. The truth is, you're not alone. Others have traveled this road. What follows is an outline of the most challenging behaviors exhibited by those with dementia, their potential causes, and how to use the 4 D's of Dementia Care to make your journey easier.

Repetitive Questions

Common caregiver questions and concerns:

- How do I deal with my loved one when they repeat the same questions?
- Responding to my loved one's repetitive questions is exhausting. What can I do?
- How do I get my loved one to stop asking the same questions?

When your loved one repeats the same thing over and over again, your first instinct may be to dismiss them, ignore them, argue with them, debate them, or correct them. But doing so can cause your loved one to get angry, agitated, upset, or paranoid. Those feelings can lead to their becoming suspicious or distrustful, which makes caring for them much more difficult.

Key Points

It's important to remember that:

- The disease is causing them to behave this way.
- They are not trying to annoy you.
- Dismissing, arguing, confronting, explaining, and correcting your loved one can make things worse for both of you. They can get defensive, angry, confused, and frustrated. Keep in mind that they aren't able to control what they think, say, and do.

- They may have moments of clarity, but those moments are fleeting. Don't be fooled by this. Researchers don't know why this happens, but these moments are temporary and beyond their control.
- It's okay to take a timeout. It's hard to stay calm and refrain from being abrupt with your loved one when you've been asked the same questions a dozen times. You're human, and your patience wears thin. You're allowed to take a few moments to compose yourself by texting with a friend, going outside, or screaming into a pillow. That short break might be just enough time to collect yourself and better deal with their repetitive questions.

Potential Causes

Your loved one may ask repetitive questions because:

- They have short-term memory loss and don't realize they're repeating themselves.
- They're reliving past events that have significant meaning to them.
- They're saying something that is important to them, that they're concerned about, or that they're afraid of.
- They're in physical discomfort or pain and can't articulate their needs.
- They're confused about the day or time.
- They're trying to initiate conversation.

- They aren't satisfied with your response.
- They're feeling distant from you.
- They're in an unfamiliar environment.
- There has been a change in their routine.
- They're bored.
- They want reassurance.
- They need to feel connected to you.
- They need to have a sense of purpose.

Implementing the 4 D's for Repetitive Questioning

Detach: People living with dementia aren't aware that they are repeating themselves. When you take a step back and recognize that it's the disease talking, it becomes easier to refrain from reacting and instead find a solution that satisfies your loved one and makes life easier for you.

For example, every morning when Tracy wakes up, she asks Emma, "What can I do for you today?" This repetitiveness annoys Emma, who often says, "Please go back to bed so I can sleep a little longer. Stop bothering me." Emma's response agitates her mother, who then becomes restless. This causes both of them to start the day on the wrong foot. Realizing that her mother can't control the questioning, Emma learns to detach from the situation and instead comes up with a plan for dealing with it.

Emma's plan is that, every evening before she goes to bed, she puts something out for her mother to do first thing in the morning. Emma comes up with seven different tasks, one for each morning of the week. On Sunday night, Emma leaves clothes hanging over the chairs in the kitchen. On Monday morning, when her mother asks, "What can I do for you today?" Emma is prepared and responds by telling her to put the clothes in the washer. On Monday evening, Emma leaves wash rags out on the kitchen counter. On Tuesday morning, Emma responds to her mother's question by telling her to clean the kitchen counter and table. By implementing her plan, Emma can get an extra 30 to 45 minutes of sleep each morning.

Your response to your loved one's repetitive questions depends upon their cognitive functioning. Many times, a verbal response is sufficient. What's most important is acknowledging that you hear their question and providing them with an answer that satisfies or comforts them.

Document: Repetitive questions serve a purpose; try to identify why your loved one repeats the same question. Listen to their exact words and see if you can pinpoint the purpose of their question. Their questions may have themes, such as:

- Something of importance to them: "When are we going to the bank? I need to get money."
- A concern or worry: "When is Roberta coming over? I haven't heard from Roberta. I need to call her."
- A fear: "Where are you going?" "What are you doing?" "When are you coming back?"
- Something memorable: "When are we going to Florida to see Jonathan? He's waiting for us."
- Reliving a past trauma: "We need to get out of here! They're coming to get us! We need to leave now!"

Pay attention to the emotion being expressed. When your loved one repeats a question, try to guess what they're feeling. Don't worry if you guess wrong. Depending on how advanced the dementia is, if you're wrong, your loved one may correct you, and you'll have a better understanding of how best to respond to them.

As your loved one's brain deteriorates, they lose the ability to communicate their needs. Instead, they repeat the same questions. In your documentation, focus on your loved one's underlying need by considering:

- Are they afraid or concerned?
- Does the questioning occur at a specific time of day?
- Are the questions related to something in the past?
- Are the questions always about the same person or event?
- Are the questions about a future event?

Diffuse: If you can identify the need behind the repetitive question, you can provide your loved one with a reassuring or comforting response. This may involve a direct statement, such as Emma's response to Tracy's question, "What can I do for you today?" Or, it may involve therapeutic acts of kindness — telling your loved one something that isn't true or withholding information to prevent them from getting upset, angry, agitated, or anxious. For example, when Tracy asks Emma where her deceased father is, she might say, "I'm not sure where he is. Is there something you'd like me to tell him?" Or, Emma might make a blanket statement, such as, "I know you miss Daddy. I do, too." The key is to keep your responses short and simple. It conserves your energy and makes it easier for your loved one to understand, thereby lessening their frustration.

Diffusing repetitive questions involves providing reassuring and comforting responses, but it can take a few tries to figure out what works. Be creative, and don't give up. The process of trial and error is essential.

Distract: Once you diffuse the situation by providing a comforting response, immediately redirect your loved one's attention. Sometimes, the only way to get someone living with dementia to stop repeating themselves is by distracting them or engaging them in an enjoyable activity. You might offer them their favorite snack or beverage, invite them to share a story, or ask them to help you with a task. Ideas for activities are outlined in the PACE "Acknowledge Their Reality" section.

Bathing

Common caregiver questions and concerns:

- My loved one refuses to bathe. What should I do?
- It's difficult to get my loved one to shower, and it triggers anxiety for me. Is there a way to make this easier for both of us?
- Should I force my loved one to shower?

For most of us, bathing or showering is intensely personal. Imagine having someone in the bathroom trying to assist you. You might feel vulnerable, exposed, embarrassed, uncomfortable, or even humiliated — and you don't have dementia. As dementia progresses, your loved one may become very resistant to bathing. In fact, bathing can become one of the most frustrating and difficult personal care activities you encounter.

Key Points

It's important to remember:

- Anything that requires many steps can be challenging for someone with dementia. They may not be able to process the information nor recall or follow steps in succession. Bathing is a prime example of this challenge. It requires putting out a clean towel, removing your clothes, gathering fresh clothes, entering the bathroom, turning on the water, making sure the water is at a comfortable temperature, getting into the shower, locating the shampoo, locating the soap, washing your hair, cleaning all of your body parts, rinsing off, turning off the water, getting out of the shower, drying off, putting on clean clothes, and drying your hair. So many steps can be overwhelming and exhausting for someone with dementia.

- People with dementia are very sensitive to water temperature and water pressure, so set your water heater to a lower temperature.

- The process is easier if the bathroom has safety features. To make the bathroom safer, you can use non-skid floor mats, install grab bars, and use a bath bench. Don't leave your loved one alone in the bathroom.

- If your loved one is comfortable, they may be more cooperative. To make the bathroom more comfortable for your loved one, use a handheld shower attachment. Have a comfortable place for your loved one to sit while they dry off and get dressed.

- Use products with non-breakable containers and keep sharp objects like tweezers and scissors out of reach.

- Your loved one may no longer understand how mirrors work and jump to the conclusion that someone is in the bathroom with them. If this happens, remove mirrors from the bathroom or cover them with sheets.

- If it's a battle, don't try to force your loved one to bathe every day. The goal is to get them in a routine of bathing once or twice a week.

Potential Causes

Your loved one may resist bathing because:

- They're afraid of falling.
- They're frustrated because they lose track of the steps involved.
- They don't understand or remember the reason for bathing.
- They don't remember how to bathe.
- They perceive the intimate experience of bathing as unpleasant or intrusive.
- They don't have the energy or stamina that bathing requires.
- Having help makes them feel exposed and vulnerable.
- The bathroom or floor is too hot or cold.
- The water is too hot or cold.
- They resent the loss of independence and privacy.
- They don't know how to turn the handles on and off.
- They think they will go down the drain with the water.
- They think you're going to force them to lay down in the shower or tub, and they won't be able to get up.

Implementing the 4 D's for Bathing

Detach: Try not to take your loved one's refusal to bathe personally. Instead of viewing it through a lens of defiance, understand that their refusal is a reflection of their brain malfunctioning. Try to remain flexible, patient, and calm. If you get frustrated or angry, walk away and try again another time. Don't try to force your loved one to bathe.

To establish trust, validate your loved one's feelings, fears, or concerns. For example, you might say, "Thank you for letting me know you don't want to shower right now. Maybe we can do it later." Or, you might say, "Sometimes, I don't like to take showers either. What if we do it together?"

Document: Try to figure out your loved one's reason for refusing to bathe. Perhaps they don't know how to shower. Maybe they can't process what you're asking them to do. It could be that there are too many steps involved or that the words "bath" and "shower" trigger a negative reaction.

Write down your observations and ideas, such as:

- What do you notice about your loved one when you try to get them to bathe?
- What do they say and do when you try to get them to bathe?
- What is the most challenging or frustrating part of trying to get them to bathe?
- How can you simplify the process?
- What can make the experience more fun and less overwhelming?

- What does your loved one like to do when they bathe?
- What do they hate most about bathing?
- What time of day is your loved one most likely and least likely to bathe?
- How can you make the process more comfortable and safer for your loved one?

Diffuse: The first step in diffusing bathing challenges is simplification. These strategies can help:

- Establish a routine and be as consistent as possible. Try to mimic the bathing routine and time of day your loved one followed prior to getting dementia.

- Pay attention to your body language, tone of voice, and facial expressions. Try to be upbeat and enthusiastic. Avoid arguing or forcing your bathing preferences onto them. One of the biggest traps is trying to convince your loved one to bathe the way you want them to bathe. Your way is not necessarily the best way for your loved one. Your way may be too complicated, difficult, or frustrating for them. They may not comprehend what you want them to do, or you may be asking them to do too many things at one time.

- Change your vocabulary. Try to avoid saying the word "shower" or "bath" and instead refer to "going to the spa," "getting a spa treatment," or "going into the locker room." Replace the word "you" with the word "we" or "us." For example, you might say, "It's time for us to wash up," "I look forward to doing this fun activity with you," "It's that time of day when we get cleaned up," or "It's time for us to pamper ourselves."

- Prepare the bathroom in advance. Have large towels available so you can cover your loved one's body for privacy and keep them warm. Have the soap, shampoo, and washcloth easily accessible. Adjust the bathroom temperature to make it warm and inviting. Cover the floor with non-skid mats and sitting areas with warm towels or blankets.

- Before your loved one gets in the shower or tub, check the water temperature. Let them feel the water temperature so they have a sense of control over the process and make sure it's not too hot or cold for them.

- Clearly communicate. Bathing involves many steps from beginning to end. Don't assume your loved one understands and remembers what to do. Take the steps one at a time and allow your loved one to participate in the process. They may need both visual and physical cues. Make eye contact, speak slowly, and demonstrate what they need to do. This may involve tag teaming the bathing experience. For example, your loved one washes your arm, and you wash their arm.

- Bathe together. Bathing can be a terrifying experience for a person with dementia, so they might feel safer if you bathe together. For example, if you're bathing together, your loved one's fear of falling can lessen considerably.

- Pick your battles. Let your loved one shower with their underclothes on if that's going to expedite bathing. Once their undergarments get wet, they may be more inclined to take the wet clothes off. Or, drape towels over your loved one's body, so they don't feel exposed, or cover their lower body with a towel while cleaning their upper body and vice versa.

- Take the path of least resistance. Use non-rinse products like dry shampoo, wash their hair in the sink, or take your loved one to a hairstylist or barber.

- Wash your loved one's less vulnerable areas first and slowly work your way toward cleaning their private parts. For example, start with getting their feet wet, so they get used to the water touching their body.

- Be gentle when drying off your loved one.

- Let your loved one hold on to something – a washcloth, soap, or shampoo. Give them a sense of participation.

- Have them sit on a bath bench or shower chair to make them feel safer and more comfortable.

- Fill plastic cups with water and let them pour the water down their back or arms and legs to rinse off the soap instead of using the handheld shower.

- When in doubt, put yourself in your loved one's shoes. Think of ways you would want to be approached and what you would like someone's tone of voice and facial expressions to be. Try doing those things to make your loved one feel safer and more secure.

Distract: Making the bathing experience fun and inviting minimizes fear and provides a welcome distraction. These strategies can help:

- Combine bathing with something else that is fun. Play music, encourage your loved one to share a favorite story, or play patty-cake while bathing.

- Create a reward system. Offer a treat after each bath. For example, you might say, "After we're done, we're going to have hamburgers and fries."

- Support their independence. Allow your loved one to do as much as possible. In the earlier stages of dementia, your loved one may only need a reminder to bathe. As the disease progresses, they will require more assistance.

- Make up a game. This takes the focus off of the act of bathing and instead places it on the game.

Toileting

As dementia progresses, toileting becomes a common problem. What we've taken for granted our entire lives becomes very confusing and complicated for a person with dementia. They lose their ability to recognize and use what was once familiar. We know what a toilet is and when to use it. Your loved one may no longer know what a toilet is, let alone its purpose.

Key Points

It's important to remember:

- Sometimes, people with dementia walk away from the toilet without pulling their pants up, which is a fall hazard.

- Provide your loved one with as much privacy as possible. Downplay having to assist them by combining toileting with another activity.

- Your loved one may not be able to see a white toilet seat, so consider switching to a colored toilet seat.

- They may not know or be able to communicate that they've soiled themselves.

- Toileting is very personal for people who don't have dementia. This doesn't change because someone has dementia.

Potential Causes

Your loved one may have issues toileting because:

- They may not recognize what the toilet is for and how to use it.

- They don't want any help due to embarrassment or fear that you're going to hurt them.

- Their brain doesn't signal the urge to use the bathroom; therefore, they don't attempt to go to the bathroom.

- They have poor depth perception and a fear of falling.

- They can't see the toilet.

- They don't have enough strength or energy to get on and off the toilet.

Implementing the 4 D's for Toileting

Detach: Your loved one's toileting issues are a result of dementia. Although toileting issues become very taxing, it's important to anticipate the problem and create a plan for dealing with it. Pay attention to your facial expressions, tone of voice, and body language. Although it may be challenging, try to smile, show enthusiasm, and be complimentary.

Document: Observe and write down your loved one's toileting behaviors with the intent of identifying patterns, causes, or triggers. Ask yourself:

- How often do accidents occur?

- Where do accidents occur?
- What do they have the most difficulty doing: finding the bathroom, knowing where the toilet is, knowing what the toilet is for, sitting on the toilet, or getting off the toilet?
- How often do they need to go to the bathroom?
- When do they usually urinate or defecate?
- Can they see where the toilet is?
- Are they afraid to sit on the toilet?
- Is the toilet seat too low, too cold, or too hard?
- What are the signs that they need to go to the bathroom? Common signals include fidgeting; pulling or tugging on their clothes; getting upset, agitated, or irritable; and going into a corner of the room.

Diffuse: Normalize their experience to the greatest extent possible. These strategies can help:

- Validate that they had an accident and be empathetic. You might say, "Oops, we missed the target. Let's clean it up, and maybe we'll have better luck next time." While with your loved one, try to downplay the frustration you feel about your loved one making a mess and creating more work for you. However, make sure you have someone to talk to about how stressful and frustrating this is.
- Create a toileting schedule. Plan on taking your loved one to the bathroom every two to three hours or after every meal and before bedtime.

- Decrease the volume of liquids by early evening. Keep in mind, though, that dehydration can lead to a urinary tract infection. Make sure that they stay hydrated throughout the day.
- Avoid caffeine and alcohol, as they can increase urination urgency.
- Choose clothing that is easy to remove, such as pants with an elastic waistband. If your loved one needs help removing their clothes, do so slowly. You may have to remind them or demonstrate how to pull their pants down.
- Plug in a nightlight near the bedroom door, down the hallway to the bathroom, and in the bathroom. Remove any clutter from the hallway.
- Remove or hide anything that could be mistaken for a toilet, such as planters, pots, and wastebaskets.
- Buy adult underwear (don't call them diapers) and put plenty of protective padding on the bed. If they soil themselves, you can change the wet bedding more easily.
- Don't rush your loved one. They may need time to empty their bowels and bladder. It may take them a while to get started. Step outside the bathroom door and wait for them to ensure they are safe.
- Give your loved one toilet paper. You may need to help them start. If you're doing the wiping, wipes may be easier than toilet paper.
- Use visual cues. Put up pictures of how to use the toilet on the wall or post a note or sign on the bathroom door that

reads "Bathroom" or "Restroom." These cues tell them what the room is, what the toilet is, and how to use it. Make sure they can see the toilet by leaving the bathroom door open.

- Keep a urinal or portable commode near the bed.
- Install grab bars next to the toilet.
- Use a raised toilet seat or a toilet support rail.

Distract: Reframe your loved one's bathroom experience. These strategies can help:

- Switch up your bathroom communication. Instead of referring to the "bathroom," use phrases like "restroom," "pit stop," "spa," "powder room," or "locker room." Reference the restroom as a place where you can pamper yourself or take care of personal needs. You can say, "Let's take a pit stop before we eat dinner," or "Before the movie begins, let's go freshen up."

- Create a positive association between toileting and doing something pleasurable afterward. For example, you can say, "Let's make a pit stop before we have frozen yogurt," and then serve the frozen yogurt immediately after they finish using the bathroom.

- Sing one song with your loved one before they use the toilet and a different song after using the toilet.

- If an accident happens, deal with it and immediately redirect their attention to something enjoyable. You always want to minimize their embarrassment.

Incontinence

As parents, we're experienced in dealing with our toddlers' lack of bladder and bowel control. Once our children are potty trained, we don't give it another thought — until our adult loved one doesn't have control over their bladder or bowels. In the later stages of Alzheimer's and other types of dementia, many people experience incontinence. Your response to their incontinence can help your loved one retain their dignity.

Key Points

It's important to remember:

- Incontinence is not always caused by dementia. If your loved one has recently started to have accidents, first check with their doctor to see if there could be a medical cause.

- As the brain declines, its signaling and message system starts failing. As a result, a person with dementia may have accidents more frequently and get confused about where and when to urinate and defecate.

- As dementia progresses, a person's mobility and ability to react quickly lessen, and they can't get to the bathroom in time.

Potential Causes

Your loved one may have issues with incontinence because:

- The messaging between the brain and the bladder or bowels doesn't connect.

- They aren't aware that they have a full bladder or bowels.
- They don't have the control needed to empty their bladder or bowels.
- They forget where the bathroom is located.
- They are experiencing the side effects of medications, such as diuretics, sleeping pills, or anxiety-reducing drugs.
- Their clothing is too tight or difficult to remove.
- They are constipated.
- They are drinking soda, coffee, tea, or alcohol, which act as diuretics and can increase urination.
- A physical issue – such as a urinary tract infection, diabetes, or diarrhea – may lead to an accident before they can reach the bathroom.

Implementing the 4 D's for Incontinence

Detach: Incontinence is something that occurs as a result of dementia or another physical condition. It's not something your loved one can control. Managing your loved one's incontinence is incredibly exhausting. Reminding yourself that the disease is causing incontinence can help you keep it in perspective and be supportive.

Document: Observe and write down your loved one's incontinence issues with the intent of trying to identify any patterns, causes, or triggers. Ask yourself these questions about their incontinence:

- When do accidents occur? Are they random, or is there a pattern?

- Did the incontinence begin suddenly?
- How long has incontinence been happening?
- When your loved one intends to use the bathroom, do they go in an unusual place like the planter box, the corner of a room, or on top of a footstool?
- Do you notice odd behavior before your loved one has an accident?
- Does your loved one say anything before they have an accident?
- Does it happen after your loved one drinks certain liquids or eats certain foods?
- How late does your loved one drink fluids?
- Does your loved one argue or exhibit frustration, agitation, anxiety, or anger before an accident?
- Have there been any changes to your loved one's medications?
- Before an accident, does your loved one exhibit any warning signs that they need to use the bathroom?

Diffuse: While it's easier said than done, it's important not to yell at or scold your loved one for having accidents. Instead, do what you can to help alleviate their embarrassment or anxiety. These strategies may help prevent accidents:

- Limit the types and kinds of fluids that can lead to incontinence. Limit fluids before bedtime, but do not withhold all fluids. Withholding fluids can cause dehydration, a urinary tract infection, increased incontinence, or agitation.

- Be on the lookout for signs that your loved one may need to use the bathroom. These signs include restlessness, pulling or tugging on clothes, or moving into a corner. Understanding the signs can help you head off accidents before they happen.

- Use adult words, such as "restroom" or "toilet," rather than baby talk, which infantilizes an adult who deserves dignity and respect.

- Avoid calling padded undergarments "diapers." Instead, call them "adult underwear," "protective pads," or "briefs." Calling undergarments "diapers" can be insulting and demeaning.

- Learn your loved one's language for needing to use the bathroom. They may say, "I can't find the bowl," or "Where is my chair?" or "I need to go into that other room." As the disease progresses, it becomes very difficult for your loved one to identify or communicate their need to use the bathroom.

- Keep cleaning supplies and rags on hand to deal with accidents.

- Make an incontinence travel kit. Stock it with underwear or adult briefs, wipes, a pair of pants, extra pads, and socks.

- Consider using waterproof mattress covers, incontinence pads for furniture, and absorbent padded undergarments.

- Give your loved one extra time in the bathroom.

- Stimulate urination by turning on the sink or tub.
- Check the toilet to see if they have urinated or have had a bowel movement.

Distract: After an accident, minimize your loved one's embarrassment by distracting them. For example, talk to them about something you're looking forward to doing with them, offer to give them a treat once everything is cleaned up, or engage them in a helper activity or an activity you know they enjoy.

You may enjoy a distraction as well. For example, while you're cleaning up, you may want to turn on music or listen to a podcast. Or, you may have a calming phrase that reinforces the fantastic job you're doing in taking care of your loved one. For example, you might say to yourself, "This is a messy job in more ways than one," or "Little did I know I would literally be cleaning up my loved one's messes," or "I need to pat myself on the back because this sure isn't what I signed up for. The things we do for love."

Apathy

Apathy is one of the most common behavioral disturbances associated with dementia. Apathy is a loss of motivation that can surface in several ways:

- Difficulty in starting or completing a task – even activities they once enjoyed;
- Lack of motivation or desire to do anything, such as daily routines;
- Low energy, which can manifest as sleeping more, being tired all of the time, or staring out of the window;
- Diminished emotions, which can appear as a lack of concern, interest, or enthusiasm; or a lack of willingness to converse or engage in social activities;
- Blunt affect, such as having no reaction or emotional response to either good or bad events; and
- No curiosity about what is happening around them and no desire to share new ideas.

Key Points

It's important to remember:

- Apathy can be a sign of depression, but can also occur separately from depression.
- Initially, those with dementia want to avoid judgment and embarrassment, so they may withdraw from people and activities.

- As they transition from mild to moderate or from moderate to severe dementia, your loved one may not be able to initiate interactions or activities.

- Withdrawing or shutting down can change your loved one's personality. This drifting away can profoundly affect you.

- Apathy makes your loved one's life less enjoyable and increases your stress.

- Apathy can be incredibly frustrating because it increases your feelings of loneliness and isolation. Watching your loved one withdraw from family, friends, social gatherings, and other activities can also be distressing.

Potential Causes

Your loved one may experience apathy because:

- The brain's frontal lobe – the part responsible for planning, judgment, and insight – deteriorates as dementia progresses.

- The brain damage from dementia causes changes in brain chemicals and brain function.

- The brain is less active and isn't consistently stimulated by and engaged in activities, so it starts to shut down.

Implementing the 4 D's for Apathy

Detach: Don't take it personally when your loved one isn't interested in following your suggestions. They aren't intentionally ignoring you or rejecting you. Their brain cells are deteriorating, and this is affecting their ability to engage in conversation and activities. This is not something they can control.

Still, it is exhausting and frustrating to care for a loved one with apathy, and you may get impatient or upset. This is entirely normal. Throughout the day, try to take regular breaks and do something you enjoy. Consider joining a support group, seeing a counselor, or talking to a good friend. The more support you receive, the less alone you will feel.

Document: Apathy is often confused with depression. Many people with depression also display apathetic behaviors. It can be difficult to recognize the difference between apathy and depression. To complicate matters, signs of depression can mimic symptoms of dementia.

The signs of depression include:

- Tearfulness or feelings of sadness;
- Feelings of hopelessness;
- Feeling worthless;
- Suicidal thoughts;
- Recurring thoughts of death; and
- Angry outbursts or irritability.

In the absence of other symptoms of depression, your loved one may be exhibiting apathy if:

- They know how to participate in an activity but don't want to do it.
- They show no interest in doing things.
- They have an "I couldn't care less" attitude about what goes on around them.
- They lack initiative.
- They lack the desire to be with you or with other people.

If you believe your loved one is suffering from depression, speak to their doctor. This is especially urgent if your loved one says they don't want to live anymore or want to kill themselves. Sometimes, people with dementia say these things to express their fears or frustrations over losing control, but they don't intend to kill themselves. It can be difficult to determine whether this is conscious planning or dementia talk; either way, it needs to be taken seriously.

Diffuse: Keeping your loved one engaged and active helps slow their cognitive decline. Here are strategies to counteract the apathy that often accompanies dementia:

- Set up a straightforward daily routine that encourages your loved one to engage in a series of activities that eventually become habitual.
- Engage your loved one in tasks and activities that they enjoy and are meaningful to them while keeping in mind their diminished cognitive capacity.
- Plan to initiate and begin the activity with your loved one, remembering that you may need to gently prompt them and participate in the activity with them.

- Try different ways of approaching your loved one. For example, instead of asking, "Do you want to walk in the garden?" try saying, "It's time for us to walk in the garden," and have them put on their sweater and shoes. Or, suggest an activity to do together. For example, you might say, "Let's play dominoes. I love when we play dominos together."
- Make an activity more accessible to start by simplifying the task. Break it down into steps and introduce one part of the activity at a time.
- Be flexible in choosing activities that can be modified to accommodate your loved one's needs.
- Focus more on the "doing" rather than on the results.
- Engage them in things they remember by creating a scrapbook or photo album.
- Avoid activities that they can't complete or that are too difficult.
- Give your loved one a sense of belonging by making them feel important, special, and productive.
- Praise and compliment your loved one, and provide rewards for their efforts.
- Engage your loved one in passive activities, such as reading to them, watching television, or listening to music.
- Try more one-on-one interaction, such as talking, singing, holding hands, or gentle massage.

- Make changes in the environment by eliminating loud noises and avoiding large groups of people.
- Attend community-based day programs that offer activities designed to engage your loved one cognitively, physically, and socially.
- Have someone else initiate and engage your loved one in an activity.
- Hire a personal trainer experienced in dementia to develop, initiate, and monitor an exercise program. Let the trainer act as the external motivating factor for your loved one.

Distract: Providing compliments and giving your loved one with dementia a sense of purpose may counteract the passivity and loss of interest resulting from dementia. Try these communication strategies to distract your loved one:

- Use "I" messages that elicit their help and make them feel needed. For example, "I need your help. Can you please help me tape this?" Bring the item to them rather than asking them to come to you. You may need to demonstrate what you need them to do. You can also ask them to hold the item while you work on it.
- Compliment your loved one by telling them how smart they are and that you can't do the task without their help.
- Refer to what you do together as "teamwork." Say, "We make a good team," or "I'm so glad we help each other."
- Provide a reward that involves both of you before, during, or after a task.

Anger and Aggression

It can be upsetting, disturbing, and frightening when your loved one lashes out at you for no apparent reason — especially if they become angry or aggressive when you're trying to help them. It's normal to feel hurt, afraid, frustrated, or mad if, instead of appreciating your assistance, your loved one is combative, calls you names, raises their voice, throws things at you, or tries to hit, kick, or push you.

Key Points

It's important to remember:

- Your loved one has a damaged brain, which means that there may be times when they misinterpret your actions or tone of voice as threatening, confusing, or frustrating. If this happens, they may lash out at you to protect themselves.

- Rushing a person with dementia increases their stress, anxiety, and frustration, which can trigger anger or aggression.

- Before touching your loved one, approach them from the front and take a few minutes to establish rapport by chatting or telling a favorite story. This reduces surprise and confusion, both of which can lead to an outburst.

- Dementia can sometimes trigger a level of aggression that makes other people feel unsafe. Call your loved one's doctor if your loved one's anger is endangering others. When used appropriately, medication can decrease dangerous aggression and improve your and your loved one's quality of life.

- If your loved one can't calm down and is becoming a danger to you or themselves, you need help. Call a neighbor who is aware of your situation or a family member or friend who lives nearby. If you call 911 in emergency situations, make sure to tell the call center that your loved one has dementia that causes them to act aggressively. The call center must communicate to first responders that your loved one isn't behaving criminally but rather just needs help to calm down safely.
- If your loved one's aggressive behavior continues to be dangerous and interventions aren't effective, placing them in a care community may be a necessary alternative.

Potential Causes

Your loved one may become angry or aggressive due to:

Pain or Physical Discomfort
- Infection. It's not uncommon for someone with dementia to have a urinary tract infection or other infections. If your loved one can't pinpoint or verbalize why or where they hurt, they may instead exhibit aggression. If they have a pre-existing health condition, such as a bad back, arthritis, or gout, they may need pain medication.
- Bodily needs. Lack of sleep, thirst or hunger, or incontinence can cause your loved one to act out.
- Medication side effects. Side effects are common when someone with dementia takes multiple medications or their medications have changed.

Environmental Factors
- Overstimulation. Loud noises, large crowds, or being surrounded by unfamiliar people within their own home can cause anxiety, anger, and aggression.

- Time of day. Most people with dementia are more attentive during certain times of day and less alert during others. You may be able to curb aggression by coordinating your loved one's activities and appointments with times of day when they are most attentive.

- Sundown syndrome. Sundown syndrome occurs when the sun starts to set. It causes people living with dementia to have sudden emotional, behavioral, or cognitive changes.

Poor Communication
- Too much information. Lengthy or complicated explanations and instructions that are difficult to follow or being asked too many questions can overwhelm your loved one and lead them to lash out.

- Not feeling heard. Arguing with or correcting your loved one can make them angry because they feel you're not listening to them.

- Body language. People with dementia are very sensitive to body language, facial expression, and tone of voice. If you convey impatience, frustration, annoyance, or anger, it increases the chance that they will reflect those feelings back to you.

- Misunderstanding your intentions. Your loved one may not understand what you are saying or doing. They interpret your words or actions as harsh or pushy and then become fearful or defensive and turn on you. You intend to be helpful, but they might misinterpret your actions as threatening or harmful.
- You startled or scared your loved one. You may have come from behind, or you were outside their field of vision, and your presence caught them off guard.

Implementing the 4 D's for Anger and Aggression

Detach: Coping with your loved one's anger and aggression can be challenging. Keep in mind that their reactions are caused by dementia and that they may not have control over their anger. It's not your fault. Dementia may make them perceive your actions through a different lens.

It can be helpful to step into their shoes. For example, imagine that a stranger tries to take off your clothes, saying that it's time to bathe. You don't understand the concept of bathing. How do you react?

Or, imagine it's time for dinner, you're sitting comfortably in your chair, and suddenly you're told you have to get out of your chair and go into another room because it's time to eat — but you're not hungry. You likely resist getting out of your comfortable chair, but your resistance is not acceptable and is met with a demand that you get out of your chair because it's time to eat. Or, the person brings food to you and insists that you eat. How do you react?

Or, imagine you've put on your clothes for the day, not knowing that they're the same clothes you wore yesterday and that they're dirty and smelly. Someone approaches you and tells you that you need to undress and put on different clothes. They don't listen when you tell them that you don't want to change your clothes. The next thing you know, they are trying to take off your shirt and pants. How do you react?

Trying to understand your loved one's perspective can help you understand that their anger and aggression aren't personal; they're a natural reaction to how their brain processes information. This understanding can help you interact with your loved one more compassionately and effectively.

Document: Uncovering the factors contributing to your loved one's anger or aggression better prepares you if it happens again, gives you the opportunity to prevent it from happening again, and helps you figure out ways to respond and cope.

Observe and write down when your loved one acts out. The goal of writing down your observations is to see if you can identify any triggers or patterns causing them to behave this way. Think about what happened right before they reacted. Ask yourself:

- What was happening when the aggression or anger occurred?

- Was their aggression or anger a reaction to something you were doing or saying?

- Does their aggression or anger occur at a specific time of the day?

- Were you trying to get your loved one to do something they didn't want to do? If so, what was it?

- Were they reacting to your tone of voice, facial expression, or body language?
- Were you trying to rush your loved one?
- Were you touching them or going to touch them?
- Is there a physical cause behind their aggression, such as pain, medication side effects, infections, dehydration, constipation, hunger, thirst, or a toileting need?

In addition to pinpointing the cause of their outburst, pay attention to which responses help calm things down and which seem to make the situation worse. Then, reflect upon what you can do differently next time to avoid this behavior.

Diffuse: There are several ways to try and diffuse your loved one's anger and aggression, including:

Anticipate behavior. Before approaching your loved one, consider how you would want to be approached if you couldn't comprehend what is being asked of you. Anticipating your loved one's behavior might prevent or decrease the frequency of the triggering event that causes them to become angry or aggressive. However, it's important to acknowledge that your loved one may still become angry or aggressive no matter what you do. That's because they have a malfunctioning brain.

Focus on feelings. When your loved one becomes angry or aggressive, focus on their feelings, not on the facts. If there isn't an obvious cause, your loved one may be feeling frustrated, sad, scared, or lonely and doesn't know how to express those feelings adequately. Rather than focusing on the specific circumstances, try to identify and validate the feelings behind the words or actions.

For example, DeShawn and Debra are playing Rummikub, a game they've played together for years. Suddenly, Debra gets angry and accuses DeShawn of cheating. She yells at him, says she doesn't want to play with a cheater, and then gets up and walks away. During her outburst, Debra says, "I don't know why I'm so stupid. My brain isn't like it used to be. I used to beat you all the time." And then she blurts out, "I'm no good. Please don't leave me."

Shocked, DeShawn's first instinct is to defend himself and tell Debra that he isn't cheating. But he is learning to focus on her feelings. He can see from Debra's reaction that playing Rummikub reinforces her sense that something is wrong with her brain. Debra's underlying fear is that DeShawn will leave her because she's "defective." Instead of getting defensive, DeShawn responds by saying, "Sometimes, my brain doesn't feel right either, and I do things that make me feel stupid. I've learned so much from you, and I don't know what I would do without you."

Listen to understand. The emotions underlying anger and aggression in people with dementia are fear, frustration, or confusion. For example, they may be reliving a past experience and reacting as though it's happening now. They might be reacting to something you said or did. They may be reacting because they can't find what they're looking for or are doing a project that's too difficult for them. If it's safe to do so, ask them what they're feeling. Listen to their answer with both your heart and your ears. Knowing what is behind their emotion can help you come up with a response that will improve their mood.

For example, Francine has no idea what her mother, Barbara, is talking about when she screams, "How can you do this to me? I've been a good mother to you, and this is how you treat me!?" But with the help of her support group, Francine starts asking her mother questions. Their conversation goes like this:

Francine:	"I'm sorry you're so upset. What have I done to make you so mad?"
Mother:	"You just want to put me away. You don't care about me. You just want me out of your life."
Francine:	"What makes you think I don't care about you?"
Mother:	"Because you put me in this home."
Francine:	"What home?"
Mother:	"A home where I don't belong."
Francine:	"Why don't you belong here?"
Mother:	"Because it's for old people who have problems."
Francine:	"What kind of problems?"
Mother:	"They're old, and they have mental problems."

As Francine continues questioning her mother, Francine remembers that Barbara had to put her own mother into a convalescent home. Barbara has been consumed with guilt and repeats what her mother — Francine's grandmother — said. Barbara is accusing Francine of the same things her grandmother accused her mother of doing.

Once Francine realizes this, she's able to have a different conversation with her mother:

Mother:	"How can you do this to me? I've been a good mother to you, and this is how you treat me!"
Francine:	"I'm sorry you're so upset."

Mother:	"You just want to put me away. You don't care about me. You just want me out of your life."
Francine:	"I love you."
Mother:	"I don't want to be put away."
Francine:	"We're in this together. I'm not going to let anything happen to you. I'll protect you and make sure that you're safe."

Avoid arguing. While it might be tempting to try and prove your point, arguing with someone who has dementia is seldom effective. You're more likely to make them even angrier, and you won't "win."

The frustration or anger you feel is justified, which is why it's essential to establish a support network. A support group, counselor, friends, or family members can provide a safe place to talk about your experience and the emotions that surface. They can help you relieve stress and normalize what you're going through. They may even help you come up with ideas for managing your loved one's aggressive dementia behavior.

Reassure them. Take a deep breath before reacting and try to speak slowly in a soft, reassuring voice. If it's safe or appropriate, use a gentle or calming touch on their arm or shoulder to provide comfort and reassurance.

Maintain a consistent schedule. When your loved one knows what to expect, they are less anxious. Consistency gives them a sense of control and makes them feel safe, which can lessen anger and aggression.

Create a calm environment. A noisy or over-stimulating environment can trigger aggressive dementia behavior. If your loved one starts behaving aggressively, look around to see if you can quickly turn off the television, turn down the volume, or ask people to leave the room.

Remove yourself. There may be times when nothing works to calm your loved one. If that happens, make sure the environment is safe and leave the room for a few minutes. This gives each of you some space and time to calm down. When you return, there's a good chance that your loved one will have settled down and may even have forgotten that they were angry.

Choose your battles. Is what you're trying to accomplish really necessary? For example, if your loved one wants to go to bed with their shoes on, ask yourself which will be easier — letting them keep their shoes on or forcing them to take their shoes off and risking an angry reaction? If not, let it go for now and try again at a later time or a different day.

Hand them a familiar item. Holding a stuffed kitten, dog, therapeutic baby doll, or favorite photo album is sometimes calming and reassuring, thereby diffusing anger.

Call in reinforcements. If your loved one usually responds well to a family member, neighbor, or friend who lives nearby, ask them to come over to help.

Distract: After giving them space to express their feelings and listening to them, redirect their attention to something they enjoy. Music strongly impacts mood, so consider putting on their favorite music, humming a soothing tune, or playing sing-along songs. You can also offer a favorite snack, invite them to take a walk, or take them outside to look at the garden.

Shadowing

Shadowing refers to when your loved one follows you wherever you go. This is both extremely common and very challenging. Your loved one can become very anxious, fearful, agitated, or angry if they can't see or find you. You may feel that you and your loved one are joined at the hip, that you're being suffocated, that your personal space is being invaded, and that you don't get a minute to yourself. Being followed around the house all day long can be incredibly frustrating, annoying, and exhausting.

Key Points

It's important to remember:

- Your loved one isn't aware that they're shadowing you. It is an involuntary manifestation of dementia and not something your loved one does intentionally.
- You are their security blanket. As your loved one's brain deteriorates, they rely on you to feel safe. All they know is that they need to be near you and see you at all times.
- As dementia progresses, your loved one becomes highly dependent on you.

Potential Causes

Your loved one may begin shadowing you because:

- People with dementia live in a constant state of fear — fear of being alone, fear of getting lost, fear of strangers, or fear of being abandoned. Imagine that you aren't sure where you are, what to do, or how to do something that you used to be able to do. You instinctively rely on the people closest to you. You become your loved one's life preserver, and they cling to you to feel safe and secure.

- They are bored and don't have enough cognitive and physical stimulation.

- They don't have a consistent routine.

- They saw something on TV or in their environment that made them fearful.

- They have a memory of being abandoned or left somewhere.

Implementing the 4 D's for Shadowing

Detach: It's common for shadowing to occur as dementia progresses and the brain deteriorates. Your loved one's dependency on you may increase to the point that they want to know where you are every minute of the day. Some people with dementia panic if they don't see their caregiver. Your loved one may accuse you of not loving them anymore, express fear that you're going to leave them, or blame you for having an affair simply because you are out of their sight.

Dealing with shadowing is physically exhausting and emotionally draining. It can help to remind yourself that your loved one is following you around and clinging to you because they're afraid. Knowing that this is a result of fear instead of intentionally trying to annoy you can make a difference in how shadowing affects you and how you react.

Your stress level increases when you feel suffocated. When shadowing occurs, it's essential for your well-being to get breaks from your loved one. Ask family members and friends to stop by and visit, or hire in-home care or companion care so that they can distract your loved one and you can get some time to yourself. Create opportunities to take a break, even if it's for ten minutes.

Document: When shadowing occurs, write down your observations. Note the date, day of the week, time of day, when it started, and what you were doing prior to your loved one shadowing you. Try to identify patterns or triggers that cause shadowing to occur. Ask yourself:

- When did the shadowing start?
- Was there a change in medication?
- Did your loved one see something on TV that was upsetting or unsettling?
- Do they follow you around all day or only at certain times of the day?
- What do they say to you when they are following you around?
- If they can't find you, what is their reaction?
- Is there anything you say or do that is helpful?

Make adjustments based on what you discover in your documentation. For example, unless Grace is within visual range, John follows her everywhere she goes. Her husband follows her when she heads to her home office to work. He repeatedly asks, "What are you doing?" and "When are you going to be done?" Then he stands next to her and waits for her to stop. Annoyed, Grace yells, "Please go sit in the other room. I'll be out when I'm done." This response makes John agitated, and Grace is forced to stop working to help her husband calm down.

After a few weeks of documenting her observations, Grace comes to three realizations:

- She needs to keep the office door open.
- It's best to go into her office when he's taking a nap.
- He needs to be busy doing a task that helps her, giving him a sense of importance.

As a result, while Grace is working at her desk, she gives her husband papers to shred in the other room. This keeps him preoccupied. Grace even asks her friends, neighbors, and family to save their shredding and to bring it over so her husband never runs out of papers to shred.

Diffuse: You can try several strategies to lessen your loved one's need to shadow you:

Provide reassurance. Throughout the day, remind your loved one that they are safe. Repeat phrases, such as, "I'm so glad we're together," "Everything is okay," "I'm here," "I love spending time together," and "I love you." Repeating these phrases slowly and with a calm voice throughout the day may provide enough reassurance so that your loved one doesn't need to follow you every minute of the day.

You can also reinforce your verbal messages by writing down these phrases on paper and posting them on doors, walls, and cabinets throughout the house.

Establish and maintain a consistent routine. Create a routine from the time your loved one gets up until the time they go to bed. Follow the same sequence of events in the same order around the same time every day. This provides structure, predictability, and a sense of belonging and purpose. It helps your loved one feel safe and secure, and it can reduce the anxiety that contributes to shadowing.

Use a timer. If you have difficulty getting time alone, announce what you're going to do, set a timer, and tell your loved one that you will be back when the timer goes off. Let them hold the timer and watch it count down. Make sure you add enough time to allow you to accomplish what you need or want to do. Before you leave the room, reassure your loved one that you're coming right back.

Play music. Music can be soothing and comforting and can elicit positive emotions and memories while promoting a sense of connectedness. Find background music that your loved one enjoys and play it softly during the day or in the evening. It can reduce shadowing and can decrease stress, anxiety, depression, and agitation.

Encourage physical movement. The benefits of exercise are the same for people with and without dementia. Movement is especially beneficial for those who shadow, as it releases pent-up energy and can decrease anxiety. Keep in mind that the goal isn't to get their heart rate up or walk 10,000 steps. Instead, think in terms of getting your loved one's blood circulating and moving their muscles and joints. If possible, incorporate some form of exercise into their daily routine. Try chair exercises, walking, exercise bands, light hand weights, tai chi, playing catch, gardening, or even walking up and down a long hallway.

Distract: Engage your loved one in meaningful activities. When selecting activities, consider your loved one's personality, interests, former occupation, and hobbies. Keep in mind that what's meaningful for one person might not be meaningful to someone else. Here are some ideas:

Give them a project. Give your loved one a task that provides them with a sense of purpose. For example, if they were a housekeeper, have them fold or stack towels, gather laundry and put it into the washing machine, wipe down the kitchen counter, dust end tables, sort through silverware, or count napkins. If they loved to cook, give them ingredients to stir, have them set the table, or ask them to clean the pots and pans. If they were mechanically inclined, give them a simple task that requires an easy fix, such as replacing batteries in a clock, screwing on jar lids, matching up nuts and bolts, or tightening screws into pieces of wood. If they had an artistic flair, provide them with watercolors, colored pencils, colored pens, and sketch pads. If they loved to garden, give them small pots, soil, and seeds, or ask them to water the flowers in the yard. When they're occupied with a project, your loved one may feel less compelled to shadow you.

Offer favorite foods. Snacks are a wonderful distraction and can also decrease anxiety, which in turn can reduce shadowing. Choose foods that your loved one enjoys.

Watch favorite movies or TV shows. Familiar sights and sounds can have a calming effect, which in turn can decrease shadowing. Replay movies and TV shows your loved one has seen and enjoyed many times. Avoid movies and shows that are violent, action-packed, or intense. Playing the same DVD or streaming the same show every day or every few days can provide comfort and familiarity that reduces shadowing.

Create a family video recording. Ask family members and friends to record their favorite stories and memories, and then invite your loved one to watch the recording when they are shadowing you.

Create an audio recording. In your voice, record a familiar story, read sections of a book, or talk about past trips or events that were memorable. Or, record a short sequence of their favorite quotes or songs. Distract them from shadowing you by playing the recording.

Enroll them in a day program. Consider enrolling your loved one in a senior or dementia daycare program. These programs provide socialization and structure, as well as cognitive and physical stimulation. While they're enjoying the program, you can get a break from shadowing.

Sundown Syndrome

Sundown syndrome typically manifests in the middle and later stages of dementia. It occurs when the sun starts to set in the late afternoon or early evening. Sundown syndrome causes people living with dementia to have sudden emotional, behavioral, or cognitive changes. According to the Alzheimer's Association, 20 percent of people with dementia get sundown syndrome.

Key Points

It's important to remember:

- Sundowning symptoms can increase as the night wears on but usually get better by morning.

- Researchers haven't determined the causes of sundowning.

- Be flexible. Sundowning isn't the same for every person with dementia. Some experience sundowning at sunset, while others experience it at sunrise. Others may never experience sundowning symptoms at all.

- Be patient with yourself and your loved one. You can try every possible strategy, and it may not work. This isn't because you're doing something wrong, but rather due to the way dementia is affecting your loved one's mind. If non-medical interventions don't alleviate challenging sundowning behavior, you might consider putting your loved one on medication.

Potential Causes

The exact cause of sundown syndrome is unknown, but researchers hypothesize that people experience sundown syndrome due to:

- Accumulation of the sensory stimulation a person receives over the course of the day, which becomes overwhelming and stressful, causing them to act out;
- Nighttime hormonal imbalances impact a person's natural circadian rhythm;
- Fatigue;
- Anxiety caused by the inability to feel safe in the dark;
- Disorientation resulting from changes in lighting;
- Reacting to your body language, tone of voice, or non-verbal communication;
- Too much commotion in the house during the day or in the evening; or
- Low blood sugar, hunger, or thirst.

Implementing the 4 D's for Sundown Syndrome

Detach: It's important to remember that sundown syndrome isn't your fault or your loved one's fault. Try to be patient with your loved one and keep in mind:

- Your loved one senses your mood or demeanor even if you don't act annoyed or concerned.

- Sundowning behaviors can get worse when you react negatively.

- Instead of challenging your loved one or asking for explanations, keep in mind that your loved one truly believes that what is happening is real – even though you know that it's not.

- Stay calm. Speak in a soothing voice, refrain from sudden movements, and avoid spontaneously touching your loved one.

- If your loved one seems to be hallucinating or is acting paranoid, do your best to reassure them that everything is alright.

Document: Observe and keep track of your loved one's behaviors in a sundowning log. Write down the date and time of day, your loved one's symptoms and behavior, what happened just before the behavior, and what happened 24 hours prior to the behavior occurring. Also, note any aggravating factors. If you can identify potential triggers, there might be ways to minimize the frequency or intensity of sundowning behavior.

Symptoms and behaviors associated with sundowning include:

- Acting suspicious;
- Agitation;
- Anger;
- Anxiety;
- Appearing disoriented;

- Being demanding;
- Crying;
- Delusions;
- Depression;
- Emotional outbursts;
- Fear;
- Hallucinations;
- Hiding things;
- Increased confusion;
- Insomnia;
- Irritability;
- Paranoia;
- Restlessness;
- Rocking;
- Sadness;
- Stubbornness;
- Violence;
- Wandering or pacing; and
- Yelling.

These factors can aggravate sundown syndrome:

- Difficulty separating dreams from reality;
- Disruption of the regular daily schedule;
- Disruption of the person's body clock;
- Fatigue;
- Illness;
- Increasing shadows;
- Loud, violent, or quickly moving TV images; while we can tune out the TV, your loved one may think what they see on TV is real life and become agitated;
- Low or dim lighting; and
- Urinary tract infection.

Ask yourself:

- What time of day did the behavior occur?
- What were you talking about?
- Was there a specific word that triggered the behavior? For example, you might have to avoid using the word "vacation" because your loved one gets angry and hostile every time you say the word.
- What were you wearing?
- What were you watching on TV?
- Was there a lot of commotion in the house during the day or in the evening?

A sample sundowning log is on the next page.

Sundowning Log

Date / Time	Symptoms / Behavior	What Happened Just Prior?	Aggravating Factors?	Note to Self
Wednesday Nov. 15 4:30 PM	Dad was especially confused.	The wind was blowing.	He saw shadows and became agitated because he thought people were outside trying to break into the house.	Close the blinds when the wind starts blowing; turn on lights; play music and do an activity with Dad to distract him.
Friday Nov. 17 4:00 PM	Dad got up and started mumbling and wasn't making sense.	He was staring out the window with a blank look.	The sun was just starting to set.	Turn on all of the lights; give him a snack before dinner to engage him.

Download Free Resources

Scan this QR code or visit tamianastasia.com/caregivers to download the logs referenced in this book.

The exact timing and kinds of behaviors caused by sundown syndrome vary greatly from one person to another. But suppose you're able to identify the causes or circumstances that trigger a particular behavior and avoid them in the future. In that case, you may be able to minimize the frequency or intensity of your loved one's behavior. This will make your life easier.

If a physical ailment — such as a urinary tract infection, a sore, or an abscessed tooth — is the culprit, your first step is to seek medical advice. Even if a medical condition isn't apparent, your loved one's doctor can rule out underlying conditions or pharmaceutical interactions that may be contributing to sundowning.

One of the side effects of sundown syndrome is that it can prevent you and your loved one from getting adequate sleep. If your loved one has inadequate sleep, their sundowning can worsen. Changing their sleeping arrangements, such as allowing them to sleep in a different bedroom or their favorite chair, may help.

Diffuse: It may be difficult to eliminate sundowning, but you may be able to minimize or manage your loved one's behaviors as the sun starts to set. Strategies to try include:

Maintain a consistent daily routine. Try to ensure that your loved one's wake-up time, meals, activities, and bedtime occur around the same time every day and in the same order. A consistent schedule helps reduce anxiety and uncertainty.

Limit caffeine and alcohol. Avoid giving your loved one alcohol and caffeine after mid-afternoon. Those substances can interfere with your loved one's ability to sleep at night and contribute to behavioral issues, such as increased agitation, anxiety, confusion, and delusions.

Increase exposure to sunlight. Take your loved one outside for 10 to 60 minutes so they get exposure to sunlight each day. Ideally, take them outside first thing in the morning. For people with dementia, the circadian rhythm can become disrupted, and bright morning sunlight can reset their body's internal clock. In addition, it can help make them more alert, improve their functioning, and decrease their risk of falling. Sunlight is also a good source of Vitamin D.

Install a nightlight. Use a nightlight to illuminate dark spaces and reduce anxiety about unfamiliar surroundings.

Plan for quiet evenings. Avoid overloading your loved one in the evening. If they need to stay occupied, plan simple and soothing activities. An upbeat movie or stroking the family pet can help calm them, but don't argue with them if they show no interest.

Monitor TV watching. In the evening, avoid watching TV shows or movies that have a lot of action and noise. Turn off the TV to lessen background noise and overstimulation.

Increase daily activities. Someone who rests most of the day is likely to be more awake at night, which in turn disrupts the wake-sleep cycle and contributes to sundown syndrome. Sleep deprivation causes physical and mental exhaustion, which interferes with concentration, the ability to perform tasks, and learning, and increases risks for falls and accidents. Keep your loved one engaged and alert by planning a variety of activities, such as visits with friends, outings to the park, or helping with household chores.

Limit daytime napping. Limiting napping helps to increase sleepiness at night. If someone with dementia sleeps too much during the day, they can get their days and nights confused, which in turn can cause sleep deprivation for you and your loved one. Try to limit the number of naps and limit the length of each nap to one hour.

It's understandable to look forward to your loved one's nap, as it gives you a break. When you limit napping, you need to find other ways to get a break from your day-to-day responsibilities. For example, you can ask friends or family members to visit or hire companion care or an activity specialist a few times a week.

Close the curtains. Draw the curtains and blinds so the change from light to dark isn't apparent to your loved one. Keep the room well-lit to minimize shadows that can trigger sundowning.

Distract: When a person with dementia has sundown syndrome, it can be challenging to keep them physically and mentally engaged at a level they can tolerate. Pay attention to the clues they provide. Which activities do they most enjoy, and for how long? These can vary from day to day, but some activities might be more soothing later in the day.

Make a list of calming activities and begin introducing those activities in the late afternoon, as the sun begins to set. Doing so can help stave off the effects of sundown syndrome. Soothing activities for people with sundown syndrome include:

- Listening to classical or calming music;
- Looking at photographs;
- Watching a favorite movie;
- Listening to sounds of nature;
- Singing songs that rhyme;
- Playing simple and fun games;
- Drawing or coloring; and
- Simple tasks, such as folding towels, putting coins or buttons in a plastic bucket, or rolling yarn.

Overstimulation can cause increased confusion and agitation, whereas not enough stimulation can cause withdrawal. People with dementia can become extremely sensitive to their environment, so you likely need to rely on trial and error to determine the right level of stimulation for your loved one on any given day.

Wandering

It's common for people with dementia to wander and get lost. Wandering can happen at any stage of dementia; even those with a recent diagnosis are predisposed to this behavior. Even if your loved one has never before wandered, they are still at risk. It's similar to watching a toddler; they can disappear in a split second or when you least expect it. Because your loved one may forget their name and where they live, wandering is a safety issue.

The Alzheimer's Association reports that 60 percent of people with dementia will wander at some point. It's crucial to find the person as soon as possible because the survival rate for wandering people depends on how long it takes to find them. Ninety-three percent of people lost for less than 12 hours survive (meaning 1 out of 14 do not), and only 12 percent survive if lost for more than 72 hours.

Key Points

It's important to remember:

- Wandering is the term used when a person with dementia has a sudden or immediate need to do something or go somewhere, but they don't necessarily have a specific destination. They're often trying to find a person, place, or thing that is important to them, needing to flee a situation that frightens them, or feeling confused or lost and trying to find their way back home even if they are home.
- Wandering can occur at any stage of dementia.
- Wandering can occur indoors or outdoors.

- Wandering occurs because the person's brain is malfunctioning, and they often have no idea what they are doing. They're on a mission, and they're going to accomplish it.

- Most people who wander turn in the direction of their dominant hand, take the path of least resistance, and walk towards light.

- Wandering is not something you can control. You can manage it by taking preventative measures.

Potential Causes

Your loved one may be wandering due to:

- Curiosity. They are curious about something and feel the need to check it out and go exploring.

- Restlessness or excess energy. They have pent-up energy and don't know what to do with themselves.

- Confusion or disorientation. They are in an unfamiliar environment or think they're in an unfamiliar environment and are looking for a familiar or safe place to go.

- Boredom. They aren't being stimulated enough and are looking for something to do.

- Untreated pain. Because they can't communicate directly, they deal with their pain by pacing or moving around.

- Fear. They may become frightened and feel the need to flee a situation.

- Over-stimulation. They may need to remove themselves from an environment that is loud or has too many people.

- Basic needs. They might be hungry or thirsty, or they may need to go to the bathroom.

- Following past routines. They may be trying to go to work, the store, or school.

- Medication side effects. A single medicine or a combination of medications can trigger wandering.

- Weather changes. The weather can throw off the body's circadian rhythm, causing increased confusion, agitation, restlessness, and disorientation.

- Sundown syndrome. Increased confusion and stress occurring in the late afternoon and evening can lead to wandering.

Implementing the 4 D's for Wandering

Detach: Don't take wandering personally. Your loved one isn't being defiant or trying to make you angry. Wandering occurs in a split second. It's like a light switch goes on, and your loved one needs to flee. Often, they have no idea where they are going. Other times, they are on a mission to find someone or something. Either way, your loved one is intent on reaching their destination. Typically, they walk at a very brisk pace. Even if they usually shuffle or walk slowly, they walk quickly when they are in the throes of wandering.

It can be hard to believe that your loved one isn't trying to get away from you, but that's not why people with dementia wander.

The root cause is that their brain is processing information in a way that tells them they need to "do something," and that urge calls for immediate action.

Document: If your loved one hasn't shown any indication of wandering, be on the safe side and look for potential warning signs, which include:

- Taking longer to return home after driving to a familiar place or from a routine walk;
- Getting lost or forgetting how to get to and from familiar places;
- Leaving a place by mistake or actively trying to escape from a place;
- Bringing up past obligations or commitments they need to meet, such as going to work or school, visiting a deceased family member, or visiting an adult child in another city;
- Saying they want to "go home" when they are home;
- Becoming agitated, restless, or fearful;
- Anxiously pacing or walking briskly;
- Being easily distracted or very curious about what's going on around them;
- Not being able to locate common places in the house, such as their bedroom or the kitchen;
- Searching for something missing or unattainable. They may rummage through drawers, look under furniture, or

search the garage. They can look for their glasses, keys, a particular piece of clothing, tools, a note from work, or a particular book. They might search for a memento of a momentous occasion, such as an award, badge, or piece of jewelry;

- Going through the motions. They might begin a chore or hobby but not accomplish anything, such as moving dirt and pots around but not planting anything, or moving items around in a drawer but not organizing them; and

- Becoming agitated or distressed in crowded places, such as shopping malls, buses, and restaurants.

If your loved one has started wandering, keep a wandering log. Write down your observations about the circumstances surrounding their wandering. The goal is to detect triggers or patterns that precede wandering. For example, you can determine whether wandering occurs when they are in a certain mood, at a certain time of day, or when basic needs aren't met.

The next page includes a sample log that Patricia kept of Peter's wandering.

Download Free Resources

Scan this QR code or visit tamianastasia.com/caregivers to download the logs referenced in this book.

Wandering Log

Date / Time	Wandering Behavior	What Happened Just Prior?	Preventive Measures
Monday July 19 3-4 PM	Fidgeting and walking around the room.	Spoke to daughter on the phone; wanted to know where she was; couldn't find her.	Place a white board next to the daughter's photo with her name, where she lives, and when she's coming to visit.
Thursday July 22 1-2 PM	Can't sit still; wants to go outside and walk around; leaves house and starts walking down the street.	Watching a detective show on TV.	Go for a walk between 1 and 2 and don't watch detective TV shows.
Tuesday July 27 7-8 PM (after dinner)	Bolted out the door while I was washing the dishes.	Saw the neighbor in her yard.	When he sees the neighbor outside, call the neighbor to come and visit.
Wednesday August 3 1-3 AM	Woke me up 3 times, worried that lions were chasing us and we needed to get out of the house.	Before we went to bed, we were watching a nature program about lions.	Don't watch nature shows before going to bed.

The first log entry allows Patricia to see that Peter's wandering behavior occurred due to talking to his daughter. He heard her voice on the phone, but he couldn't see her and wanted to find her. Using trial and error, Patricia implements the preventative measure of placing a whiteboard next to their daughter's photo and writing on the whiteboard their daughter's name, where she lives, when she's going to call, and when she's planning to visit.

In the second log entry, Patricia sees that she and Peter watched a TV show before going to bed. During that episode, the police were chasing a suspect. Later in the evening, Peter bolts out of the house. This might have been an attempt to find the suspect in the TV show. Patricia tries to prevent this wandering behavior from occurring again by not watching TV action shows late afternoons or evenings.

In the third log entry, Peter's wandering occurred because he wanted to say hello to the neighbor he saw standing outside, but the neighbor had already gone into her home. Patricia's solution is to call the neighbor, who comes right over to visit. This prevents Peter from darting outside.

In the fourth log entry, Patricia writes down that she and Peter watched a nature show about lions before they went to bed. In the middle of the night, Peter woke her up because he thought lions were chasing them and they needed to escape. To prevent Peter from leaving the house, Patricia immediately gets up and turns on all the lights to scare the lions away and reassure her husband that they are safe.

If you're able to identify triggers or patterns, you can take preventative measures. For instance, if your loved one wanders at the same time every day, you can engage them in an activity or take them for a walk at that time of day to reduce the need to wander. If they wander when you use the bathroom, it may be because they're looking for you. An option might be to leave the door open so that, when they call your name, you can answer them and they can find you.

Diffuse: Effective communication can help prevent people who are exhibiting warning signs of wandering. For example:

- If your loved one feels lost, confused, abandoned, or disoriented, they may say they want to "go home" or "go to work." Refrain from arguing with them. Instead, provide validation and reassurance. You might say, "It's early in the morning. Why don't we have breakfast first so we don't wake everyone up?" Or, you might say, "It's a holiday, and all the offices, schools, and stores are closed."

- If your loved one is looking for a deceased relative or an adult child who is living away from home, you can say, "They are out of town and will be back in a few days. We'll go and see them when they get back." Or you might say, "She called and said she can't visit today, but she will call us later."

- If your loved one is looking for an object, reassure them that everything is okay and that the item is in a safe place. You might say, "Your watch is at the shop, and it's being fixed," or "It's in a safe place so no one can take it." If they are constantly looking for a common item, buy multiples of that item so you can pull one out and put it where they can easily find it. Commonly misplaced items are reading glasses, TV remote controls, purses, wallets, tools, shoes, jewelry, and clothing.

When communicating with your loved one, try to get them to elaborate so you can determine what they need. Encourage them to tell you more about the person or object they are looking for so you can try to figure out the reason for their urgency. Inviting them to share more information engages them and may calm them down. It also distracts them and reduces their need to go looking for what they seek. Or, if they aren't able to articulate what they need, pay attention to their body language and facial expressions to see if you can figure out what is troubling them.

Despite your best efforts, it's not always possible to prevent wandering. Yet, there are strategies you can use to decrease the likelihood of wandering, such as:

Increase physical movement. Walking, dancing, riding a stationary bike, stretching, balance exercises, or yoga may help reduce the anxiety, agitation, or restlessness that fuels the tendency to wander.

Roam in safe areas. With supervision, allow your loved one to wander in a restricted area, such as a fenced backyard, enclosed school property, or a fenced flower garden. Supervised wandering enables them to expend energy while staying safe.

Maintain a quiet environment. Too much stimulation, such as a loud television or several conversations happening at once, can cause wandering.

Prioritize cognitive stimulation. Establish and maintain a consistent daily routine that includes cognitive stimulation. Restlessness and boredom can trigger wandering.

Keep a family photo album nearby. A photo album can fulfill the desire to see a family member or a familiar sight, making it unnecessary to wander.

Post a note. If your loved one keeps looking for a family member, print out a sheet that includes the family member's photo and states they will be visiting soon. This response can be reassuring and may reduce the chance of wandering.

Install a nightlight. Your loved one's wandering might be due to dementia-related changes in vision and perception that make dark areas particularly frightening. A nightlight in your loved one's bedroom and nightlights throughout the house can reduce their fear.

Distract: After you've validated your loved one and have provided a reassuring response to their need to go somewhere or look for someone or something, it's essential to have a few distractions up your sleeve. For example, you can take them for a walk, give them a snack, participate in an activity together, turn on music, or provide them with a chore to do. This gets their mind off of where they want to go.

Safety Measures for Wandering

Wandering is more than a challenge; it can be dangerous. It can also disrupt your peace of mind. You can help ensure your loved one's safety by:

Reducing home hazards. Remove throw rugs, tuck away electrical cords, and rearrange furniture to prevent tripping. Install nightlights throughout your home and gates at the top of stairways to help prevent nighttime wandering injuries.

Installing locks on exit doors. Install either high or low door locks or slide bolts on exterior doors to reduce the chance they can leave unnoticed.

Installing wireless monitors. These devices signal when a door or window is being opened. If you already have a security system in your home, arm the system for "stay" mode.

Purchasing childproofing aids. Consider using childproof doorknob covers and door latches.

Using sensor mats. If your loved one wanders during the overnight hours, place a pressure-sensitive alarm mat on the floor next to their bed.

Camouflaging the exit doors. Cover doors so that they match the surrounding walls. Alternately, hang removable curtains over doors or put big houseplants in front of doors to prevent your loved one from recognizing an exit.

Placing stop signs. Often, people with dementia won't open a door with a large sign. Put up signs that read "DO NOT ENTER" or "STOP" on exit doors.

Posting room signs. Make signs that say "Bathroom" and "Bedroom," and place them on the corresponding doors in your home. Your loved one may forget where they are, and signs can help orient them so they don't wander.

Placing doormats. Place large black doormats in front of exit doors. People with dementia often think that dark areas are holes and refrain from walking over them. This may prevent your loved one from going to the door.

Using a tracking device. You can insert a GPS device in your loved one's shoe or pocket that sends electronic alerts about their location. If they wander, the device can help you find them quickly. Ask your police or sheriff department if they offer a locator service, such as SafetyNet or Project Lifesaver.

Never leaving them unattended. Don't leave your loved one home alone or unsupervised in a car or new environment.

Hiding the car keys. Wandering doesn't just occur on foot. Make sure car keys are well hidden.

Hiding their wallet. Sometimes, people living with dementia are creatures of habit and won't leave the house unless they have their purse or wallet. Keeping those items out of sight may keep your loved one at home.

Labeling clothes. Sew or iron ID labels containing your contact information into their clothes.

Enrolling in Safe Return. The Alzheimer's Association's Safe Return program is a nationwide identification system designed to assist families when a loved one wanders. Caregivers purchase a MedicAlert ID product and pay a registration fee for a MedicAlert membership plan. The program provides 24/7 access to a national database and an emergency response team that works with first responders.

Creating an emergency plan. If the unthinkable happens and your loved one is missing, your emergency plan can help ensure they are found quickly. Consider incorporating the following elements into your emergency plan:

- Transparent communication. Tell your neighbors that your loved one has dementia and ask them to call you if they see your loved one wandering.

- Write down contact information for those in your local support network. Keep the list handy so that you can notify your network if your loved one is missing.

- Have an ID kit prepared and readily available. Include a recent photo, a list of medications and medical conditions, and insurance information to give first responders. Add a list of potential destinations, such as former workplaces and homes, favorite restaurants, and their place of worship.

- Call 911 first. Resist the temptation to take matters into your own hands. Before embarking on a search, call first responders and tell them that the missing person has dementia.

- Know the area. In most cases, people with dementia are found within a radius of 1.5 miles. Be aware of environmental dangers, such as bodies of water, tunnels, major roadways, culverts, and tunnels.

Driving

One of the most difficult challenges caregivers face is how to deal with their loved one when they refuse to give up driving. For most of us, driving represents independence — the ability to come and go as we please. The thought of not being able to drive can be highly upsetting for the person with dementia, yet they aren't able to recognize how dangerous it is for them to be driving.

It can be hard to know when your loved one should stop driving and what to say during the difficult conversation about driving. Often, trying to reason with them can turn into a heated discussion.

Key Points

- As dementia progresses, it affects a person's ability to drive safely. Your loved one eventually needs to stop driving, as they become a safety risk to themselves and others.

- The timing for giving up driving varies from person to person. Typically, the ability to drive lessens as dementia advances.

- Some of those living with dementia willingly stop driving because they are aware and concerned about their driving skills and safety. Others may refuse to give up driving because they don't recognize the decline in their driving skills and think they are still a good driver.

- Driving can be a very emotionally charged and sensitive issue for the caregiver and the loved one. It's important to approach this topic cautiously.

Potential Causes

As the brain cells deteriorate, your loved one's ability to drive safely erodes due to:

- Memory loss. They have difficulty remembering a familiar route or destination.
- Increased confusion. It can take an exceptionally long time for your loved one to drive home from a familiar place. They may confuse the gas and brake pedals.
- Poor judgment. Problem-solving and decision-making skills decline, making them unable to maneuver or anticipate obstacles or detours in the road.
- Visual-spatial disorientation. They're unable to maintain the correct speed or distance, or stay in their lane.
- Slower reflexes. Their ability to react quickly makes it difficult to avoid collisions.
- Difficulty processing information. They're unable to understand or interpret road signage or the actions of other drivers.

Implementing the 4 D's for Driving

Detach: Once you recognize that your loved one needs to stop driving, the question becomes how to approach the issue. Discussing your loved one's ability to drive can be difficult, especially if they can't recognize their deficits and insist that they are a good driver.

While it would be wonderful to have a heart-to-heart conversation, during which they agree to stop driving, conversations about driving often lead to anger, resentment, hostility, and denial. It's essential to keep in mind that this unpleasant and hurtful exchange of words isn't about you. Your loved one may take their feelings and frustrations out on you. They're reacting to losing their independence and the unsettling thought of not being able to come and go as they please.

Ways to approach the driving issue with detachment include:

- Put yourself in their shoes. Think about how you would want to be approached about your driving. What would you like to hear?
- Prepare in advance. Think through what you want to say to your loved one. Keep a list of your observations so that you have examples to support your concerns.
- Call the doctor. Share your observations and concerns with the doctor and ask them to discuss driving with your loved one. This takes the responsibility and blame off of you. Typically, if the doctor determines that your loved one shouldn't be driving due to cognitive impairment or dementia, it's their responsibility to send a report to the DMV. Then, the DMV sends a notification to your loved one. In many cases, the DMV will require your loved one to take a written or driving test to retain their driver's license.
- Anonymously report. When you anonymously report your loved one to the DMV, the agency generally requires that your loved one take a written or driving retest, regardless of when their license expires. Consult your state's DMV website to determine the steps needed to request that someone be retested.

Document: The time when someone with dementia should stop driving varies from person to person. When you become concerned, write down your observations of your loved one's driving skills. These are some warning signs:

- Increased forgetfulness, confusion, or disorientation. Your loved one forgets where they are supposed to go, they're confused as to the day and time, or they confuse the gas and brake pedals.
- Getting lost driving to and from familiar places. For example, it may take them an hour to pick up milk when the grocery store is ten minutes down the street.
- Decreased coordination. For example, your loved one may not be able to put on their blinker and look over their shoulder at the same time.
- Easily distracted. They're unable to focus on the road.
- Difficulty scheduling appointments. They can't keep their appointments straight, miss appointments, or show up on the wrong day or at the wrong time.
- Evidence of spatial disorientation. There may be new dents and scrapes on the car. They may drive over curbs or straddle two parking spaces.
- Needing daily care or medication reminders. They may forget to take their medication or refuse to take their medication consistently.
- Poor judgment. Your loved one may drive slowly, ignore traffic signs and signals, or change lanes haphazardly.

- Heightened reactions. They may become increasingly impatient, frustrated, annoyed, angry, or confused while driving.

Diffuse: Losing the ability to drive can cause intense emotions and reactions, especially when your loved one is convinced they are a good driver. Instead of explaining why they shouldn't be driving, spend time listening to what they are telling you. Try to anticipate their reactions and prepare responses in advance. Validating and empathetic phrases include, "I'm sorry you have to go through this," "I can see how upset you are. What can I do to help you with this?" and "We'll get through this together."

Having transportation options available can help diffuse intense reactions. Be prepared to introduce alternatives to driving, and consider the impact these alternatives will have on you. For example, do you want to be responsible for all driving; can family and friends help you; or do you want to use Uber, Lyft, or a private driver?

Feelings about not being able to drive may decrease if there's not a vehicle available to drive. You can have a relative or friend "borrow" the car, or you can "lose" the keys and pretend you don't know where they are. Offer to look for them or suggest that you'll order a new set.

Alternately, you can disable the car or the key fob and then have the vehicle towed. You can store it at a friend's house until you decide what to do with the vehicle. If your loved one asks why it's taking so long to get the car back, say that the part hasn't come in yet or that the mechanic is on vacation and will work on it when they come back.

Distract: Keeping your loved one distracted from driving can be a real challenge. Try to reduce their need to drive. Here are ideas to try:

- If they are insistent on taking the written DMV test, go through the motions of helping them study for the driving test and set up a consistent study schedule.

- Begin implementing other transportation options before your loved one loses their license.

- Hire a driving coach or occupational therapist to work with them so they feel they have some control over their circumstances. Let the driving coach know your loved one has dementia so they can take precautions to practice in safe areas.

- Hire companion care or have family and friends take your loved one out.

- Decrease your loved one's desire to drive by keeping them engaged in activities they enjoy, such as gardening, chores, playing games, or watching movies.

- Have items delivered rather than going to pick them up.

- Take your loved one to a senior day center to keep them busy.

Unsafe driving is a serious and dangerous issue that needs to be addressed. There's a delicate balance between respecting your loved one's desire to drive and protecting their safety and the safety of others. While some of these suggestions involve deception, extreme measures sometimes must be taken when people living with dementia are uncooperative and unreasonable. Know that what you're doing is in their best interest and the best interest of others. As difficult as this issue is, your loved one will eventually adjust to their circumstances.

Refusing to Take Medication

Refusing to take medication is a common manifestation of dementia. As the caregiver, this can be incredibly distressing. After all, you know the importance of the medicine, but trying to explain to a person living with dementia the consequences of not taking their medication can make things worse.

Key Points

It's important to remember:

- Many seniors take multiple medications. Some may not be needed. Go over the list of medications with your loved one's doctor to see if any can be eliminated. Reducing the number of pills can also reduce the chances of your loved one refusing to take their medication.

- It's normal to get frustrated and angry when your loved one won't take their medication. Try not to take your frustration and anger out on yourself or your loved one. Instead, put your energy into trying to understand what's behind their refusal and figuring out alternatives. For example, you might be able to get the medication in liquid or powdered form and mix it in with their food.

- As the disease progresses, people with dementia may forget what medication is for and why they need it and refuse to take anything.

Potential Causes

Your loved one may refuse to take their medication because:

- They don't understand or are confused about the reason for taking the medicine.
- Refusal is a way for them to feel in control.
- They have difficulty swallowing pills.
- They don't like the medication's side effects, such as nausea, stomachache, agitation, or dizziness.
- They are distracted by other things going on around them.
- They have dental issues.
- Their brain gets overwhelmed by so many pills.
- They think the medication is harmful or poisonous.
- They don't like how the medication tastes or feels when they put it in their mouth.
- They don't like the size, color, or quantity of the medicine.

Implementing the 4 D's for Medication Refusal

Detach: Try not to take your loved one's refusal of medication personally. Remind yourself that your loved one's reaction is a symptom of dementia. This isn't something they are doing intentionally to be defiant. However, there's often an underlying reason or fear. It may not seem logical to you, but it's logical to your loved one. That said, it's normal for you to become upset and react.

Instead of reacting, try to figure out the reason behind their refusal. For example, you might say, "I can see you don't want to take your pills right now. Can you tell me why?" Pinpointing their rationale may help you find a solution.

Don't argue with their logic. Instead, think outside of the box and develop other ways to encourage them to take their medication. For example, your loved one might not like the color of their pill organizer. If you put their medicines in a differently colored pillbox, your loved one may take their medication. If the pill size is an issue, using a pill cutter to make the tablets smaller might be a solution.

Document: Keep a medication log. Track when your loved one refuses to take their medication. If you can pinpoint causes, you can find ways to increase the chance that they will consent. In your medication log, write down the date, time of day, what medications they are supposed to take, what happened when you tried to give them the medicine, the circumstances surrounding their refusal, and their reason for refusing the medication.

The next page includes a sample medication log.

Download Free Resources

Scan this QR code or visit
tamianastasia.com/caregivers
to download the logs
referenced in this book.

Medication Log

Date / Time	Medication	Reason for Not Taking	Observations
Monday April 3 9:00 AM	Morning medication	Confused; doesn't know what it is for.	I woke him up and rushed him; he didn't have enough time to wake up.
Wednesday April 5 1:00 PM	Afternoon medication	Pill too big.	I need to cut the pill in half.
Friday April 7 8:00 PM (after dinner)	Evening medication	Says, "I don't need those."	Call the medication "vitamins," and I take my medication at the same time.

To determine what may be contributing to your loved one's refusal to take their medication, ask yourself the following questions:

- Are you interrupting an activity or a TV show they are watching to give them their medication?
- Are they in a noisy room, or are there several people in the room?
- Do they believe that the medication is poison?
- Are you waking them up to give them their medication?
- When did their refusal of medication start?

- Has there been a recent medication change?
- Are they refusing to take all of their medication or some of it?
- Which medications are they willing to take?
- Which medications are they refusing?
- Are they willing to take their medications at certain times of the day but not at others?
- Are they refusing to take larger pills but willing to take smaller pills, or are they only taking pills of a particular color?
- Are they questioning what the medication is for or where you got the medication?

Diffuse: Try to stay calm and patient. If you start to get frustrated or angry, your loved one will likely sense that and also become frustrated and angry. As a result, they're less likely to cooperate. People with dementia are very sensitive to our body language, tone of voice, and facial expressions, and often mimic or imitate our behavior. In addition:

- Don't explain. Try to avoid explaining the importance or consequences of not taking their medication. Likely, they aren't going to understand what you're telling them, and trying to explain it could worsen the situation.
- Don't ramble. Use concise and clear communication to encourage your loved one to take their medication. You may also need to provide verbal and physical cues, such as

showing them how to take their pills. For example, try putting a pill in your loved one's hand and one in your hand. On the count of three, you each take your medication. Your loved one can copy your actions. Pop a vitamin or Skittle into your mouth if you don't take pills.

- Change the wording. Instead of referring to "medication" or "pills," use words such as "candy" or "vitamins."

- Don't force the issue. Don't try to force your loved one to take their medication. This could cause a physical or violent reaction. Instead, walk away and try again at a later time.

- Optimize the timing. Note the times when your loved one cooperates to determine the optimal time of day to give them medication. Consult with their doctor to see if there's flexibility in the time of day the medication can be given. If so, avoid giving them medicines during challenging times of the day. For example, if your loved one tends to get agitated or confused in the late afternoon or evening, give them their medication earlier in the day.

- Establish a consistent schedule. Consistency is essential for people living with dementia. They get used to a particular routine and sticking to the routine increases the likelihood of compliance. Give your loved one their medication around the same time every day, after the same activity, in the same room, and with the same glass or mug. For instance, you might give them the medication after breakfast, while they're sitting at the kitchen table and they have their familiar glass of water nearby.

- Reduce the quantity. Decrease the number of pills your loved one takes by omitting vitamins or supplements that their doctor hasn't recommended.

- Simplify the process. If some pills are too large or difficult for your loved one to swallow, ask the doctor or pharmacist if the medications can be prescribed in liquid form. Inquire whether the pill can be crushed and added to soft food, such as ice cream, scrambled eggs, yogurt, pudding, or applesauce. Or, use a pill cutter to reduce the size of the pill. Another option is to have your loved one take one pill at a time instead of bringing all of the medications out at once.

- Pay attention to side effects. If the pills taste bad, if they make your loved one dizzy, or if they cause stomach upset, talk to their doctor about switching to a liquid or powder, or changing the medication to another in the same family.

Distract: Sometimes, combining taking medication with another enjoyable activity can be very effective. For example, you might want to give your loved one their medication while listening to music, having a snack, or watching the birds in the backyard. The positive association may make them more amenable to taking their medication. Similarly, having your loved one share a favorite story or joke while encouraging them to take their medication may increase cooperation. People with dementia like songs or rhymes, so try coming up with a medication song or rhyme to make medication time a fun activity or a happy occasion. For example, when it's time for Peter to take his medication, Patricia sings, "Open sesame! Down the hatch it goes. You take yours. I'll take mine. We take our pills at the same time." Bob sings to Beth, "One for you, one for me, now it's time to drink our tea." You can also reward your loved one by, for example, telling them that you'll take them to their favorite restaurant after they take their medication.

Challenging behaviors — whether with personal hygiene, medication compliance, driving, or wandering — make your life as a caregiver more stressful. In the moment, it can be hard to take a step back and analyze the situation. Remember that it takes practice, that it's a process of trial and error, and that perfection isn't the goal. Making even incremental progress in decreasing the frequency or intensity of challenging behaviors can provide relief and conserve your energy.

Afterword

As a dementia consultant and educator, caregiver support group facilitator, and health and wellness counselor, I've had the privilege and honor to meet and work with hundreds of beautiful, wonderful, compassionate, and loving caregivers who are doing everything in their power to provide the best care for their loved ones. Yet, many frequently question the decisions they make on behalf of their loved ones with dementia.

Their struggle with caregiver guilt, self-doubt, and regret are both common and unjustified. This struggle inspired me to write about the caregiver's journey. I want caregivers to know they are beautiful and amazing people. I want them to have the knowledge and skills to help their loved one, but I don't want the caregiver's journey to be at the expense of their physical, mental, and emotional well-being. I want to provide an informative emotional and behavioral handbook that supports the caregiver and helps them find meaningful ways to cope with this devastating disease.

I've written this book because of my desire to:

- Let caregivers know that they're not alone;
- Increase the caregiver's self-confidence and reduce the degree of self-doubt and caregiver guilt;

- Normalize the caregiver's emotional journey;
- Validate caregivers' thoughts and feelings, whether they're perceived as positive or negative;
- Provide insights that help explain why their loved ones say and do the things they do, and why caregivers react the way they do;
- Offer strategies that can help caregivers deal with the behavioral and cognitive changes that occur throughout the dementia journey;
- Prepare caregivers for what lies ahead, including how dementia will affect their loved one and how their loved one's dementia will affect the caregiver;
- Remind and reassure caregivers that they are doing an amazing job and that their decisions are made in the best interests of their loved ones; and
- Give a gift to the caregiver.

I couldn't have written this book alone. First and foremost, I want to thank every caregiver who has allowed me to be a part of their journey. Thank you for sharing your feelings, thoughts, concerns, frustrations, challenges, blessings, tears, and laughter.

The knowledge and expertise I've accumulated are the result of working with all of the caregivers who trusted me, whether in my private practice or my support groups. I was motivated to write this book with you in mind. This book truly wouldn't have been written without you.

I owe a debt of gratitude to Randee Smith, Irene Dockins, Laura Le, and Tina Morrill for their mentoring, support, edits, and encouragement. In addition, my thanks go to Patricia E. McKeon, Ph.D., Leslie Kefer, and Sarah Jiminez for sharing their expertise when I needed additional information. More broadly, I'm forever grateful to all of my colleagues who have shared their expertise and experiences over the years and have provided wonderful services to my clients. Thank you to Sally Smith, my amazing editor. Finally, I want to thank Elizabeth A. Landsverk, MD, for sharing her expertise on medication and for helping many of my clients' loved ones living with dementia.

On behalf of your loved ones living with dementia and myself, I want to thank you for all of the love, care, and support you provide.

Dementia Resources

Caregiver Newsletters
- AgingCare: agingcare.com
- Alzheimer's Association: alz.org/e-news
- DailyCaring: dailycaring.com

Caregiver Support Groups
- Tami Anastasia: tamianastasia.com/events
- Alzheimer's Association: alz.org/help-support/community/support-groups
- Facebook groups: dailycaring.com/support-groups-for-caregivers-on-facebook

Elder Care Resources
- Aging Life Care: aginglifecare.org
- American Association of Daily Money Managers: secure.aadmm.com
- Elder Financial Protection Network: elderfinancialprotection.org

- National Academy of Elder Law Attorneys: naela.org
- Eldercare Locator: eldercare.acl.gov
- ElderCare Matters: eldercarematters.com
- Institute on Aging: ioaging.org

National Dementia Organizations
- Dementia Society of America: dementiasociety.org
- Alzheimer's Association: alz.org
- Alzheimer's Foundation of America: alzfdn.org
- Alzheimer's Research & Prevention Foundation: alzheimersprevention.org
- Bright Focus Foundation: brightfocus.org
- Lewy Body Dementia Association: lbda.org
- Parkinson's Foundation: parkinson.org
- The Association for Frontotemporal Degeneration: theaftd.org

Download Free Resources

Scan this QR code or visit tamianastasia.com/caregivers to download the logs referenced in this book and find other resources for caregivers.

About the Author

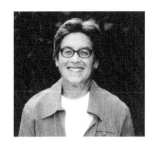

Tami Anastasia is a dementia consultant, educator, and speaker. She holds a Master of Arts in Counseling, a Certificate in Gerontology, and a Certificate in End of Life. Tami is an Evergreen Certified Dementia Care Specialist and a Certified Senior Advisor. For more than 30 years, Tami has provided counseling services, dementia guidance, emotional support, and care strategies to family and professional dementia caregivers.

In addition to her private practice, Tami facilitates dementia caregiver support groups and has partnered with agencies throughout California to conduct educational workshops, trainings, and webinars. Tami is a sought-after speaker, frequently presenting before audiences at professional meetings, senior retirement centers, memory care and assisted living communities, health and wellness conferences, colleges and universities, and public health organizations.

Tami hosted TAMS Health and Wellness on the VoiceAmerica Health and Wellness Channel, and is the author of the groundbreaking exercise book, *Toward a Magnificent Self: The Exercise Book for Every Body,* focused on the psychology of exercise habits and realistic solutions to overcoming exercise barriers.

For more information, visit tamianastasia.com

Made in the USA
Monee, IL
06 February 2023

27258674R00162